Different Areas of Physiotherapy

Edited by Mintaze Kerem Gunel

Published in London, United Kingdom

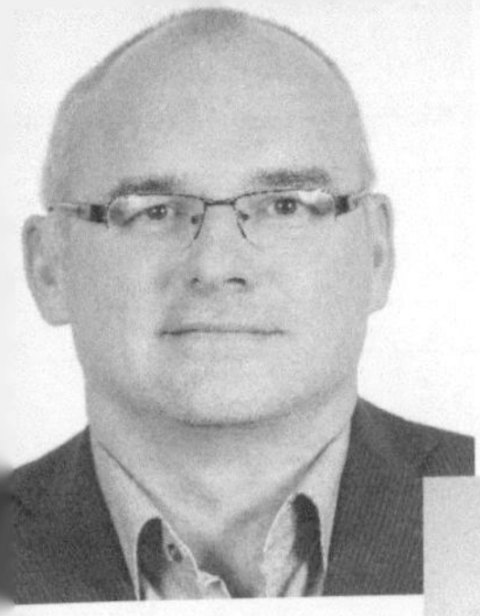
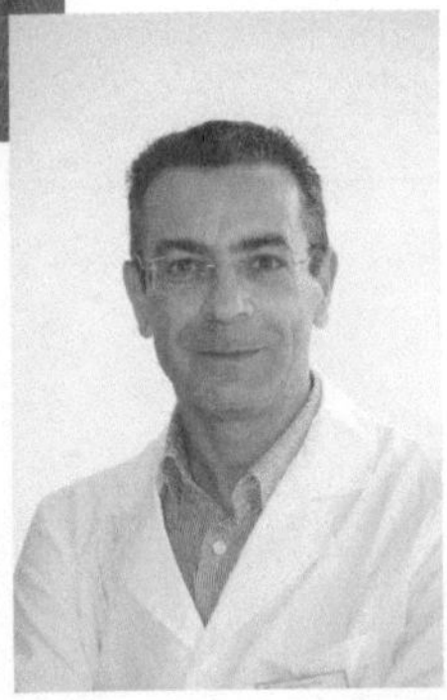
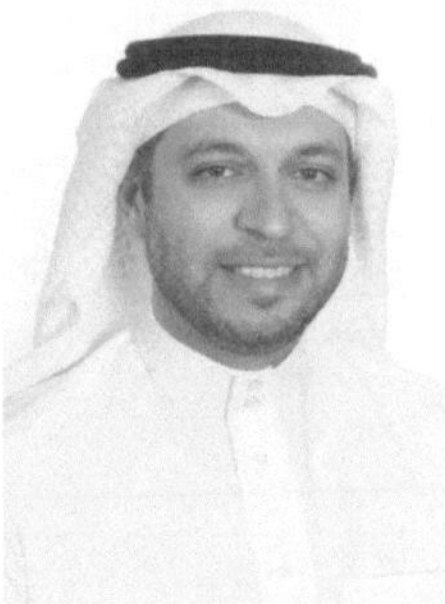
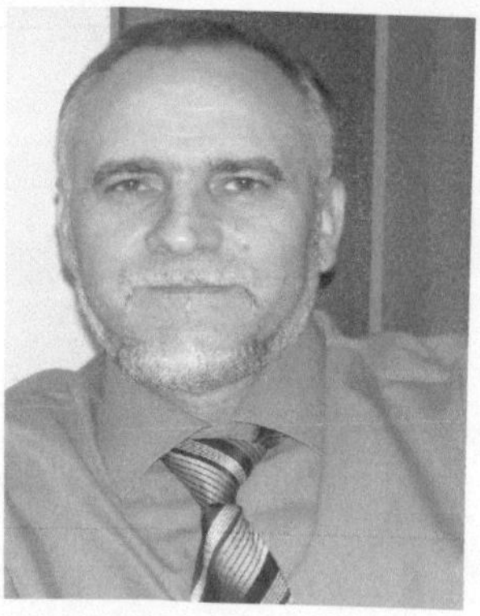
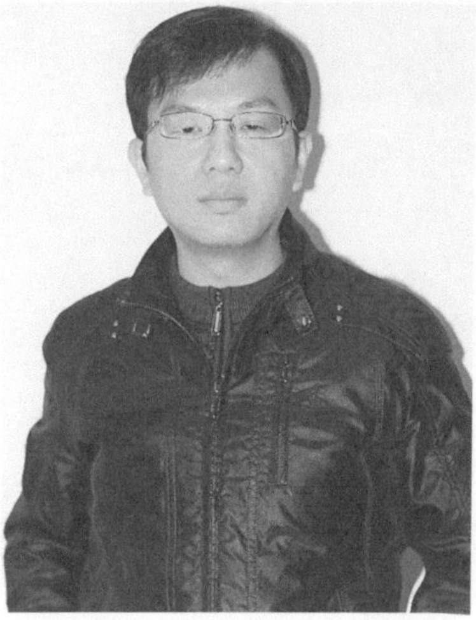
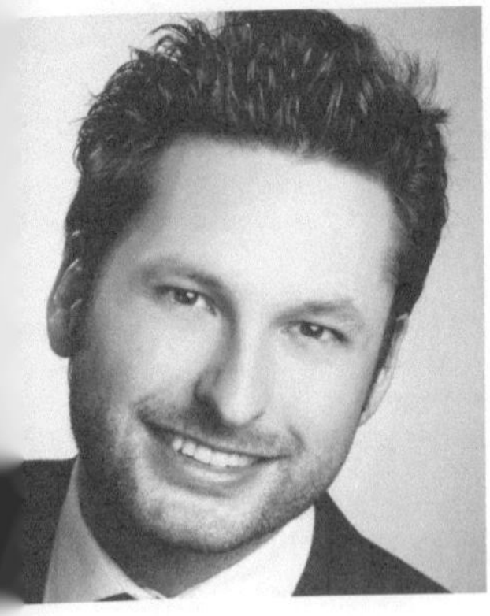
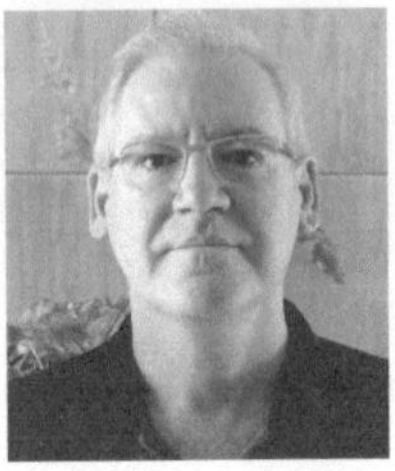

IntechOpen

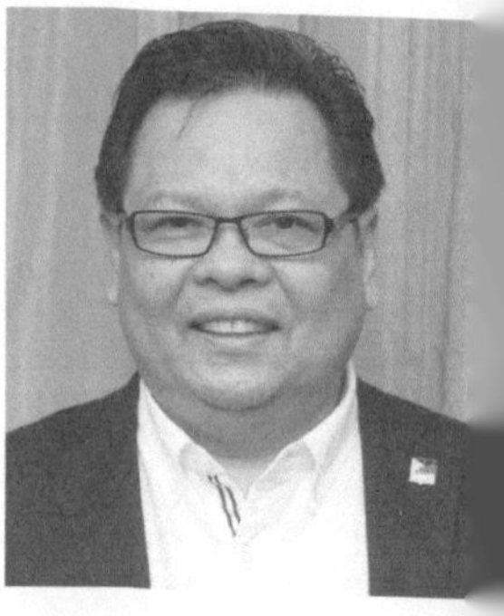
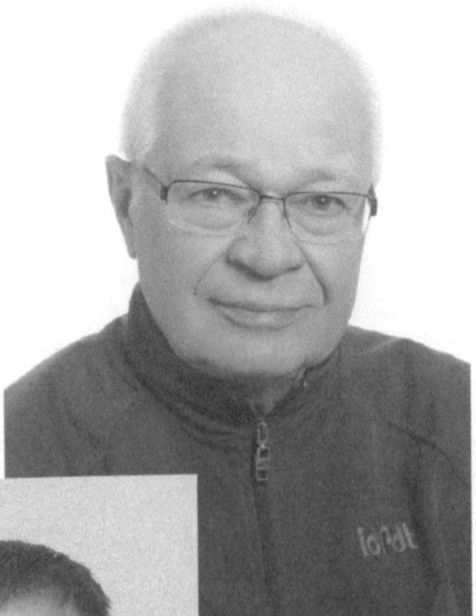
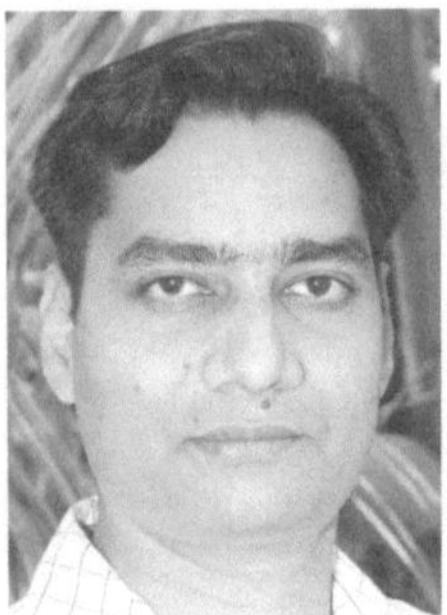
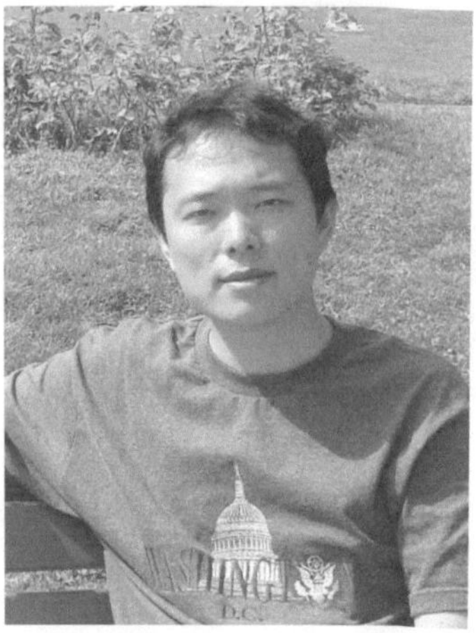
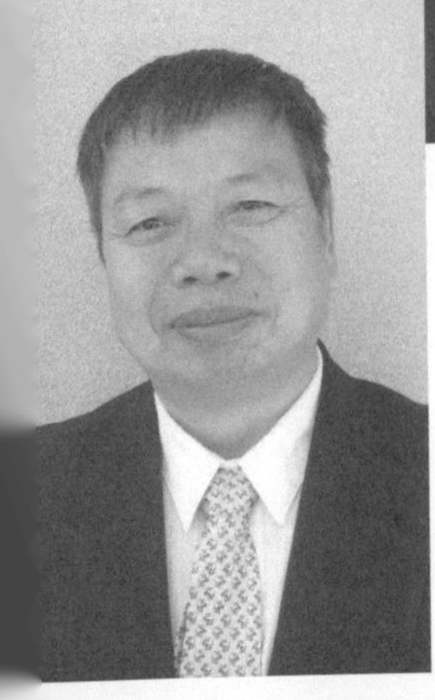
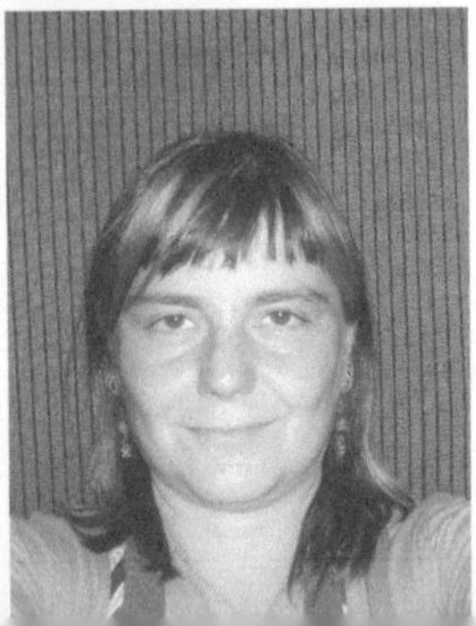

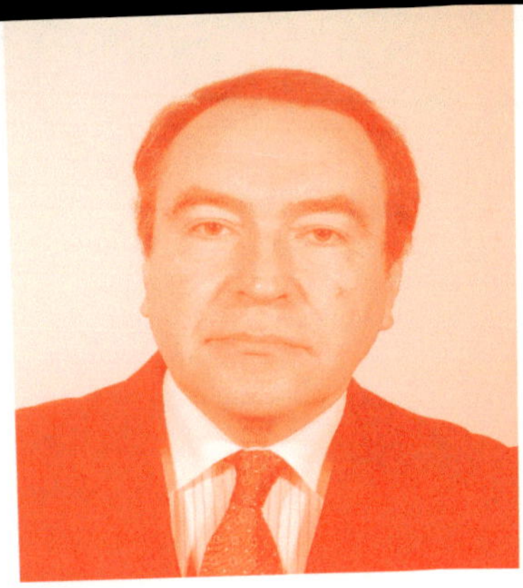
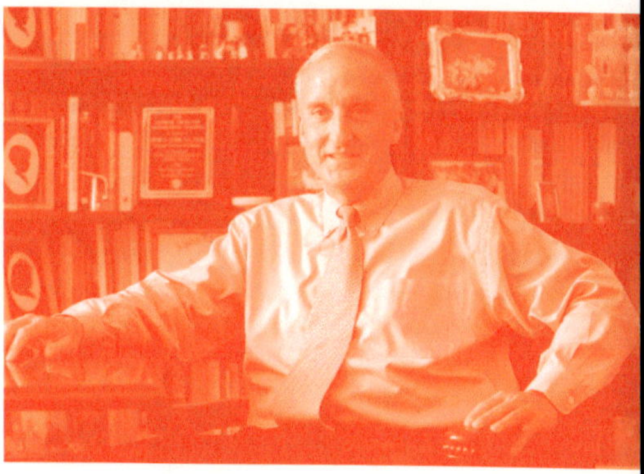
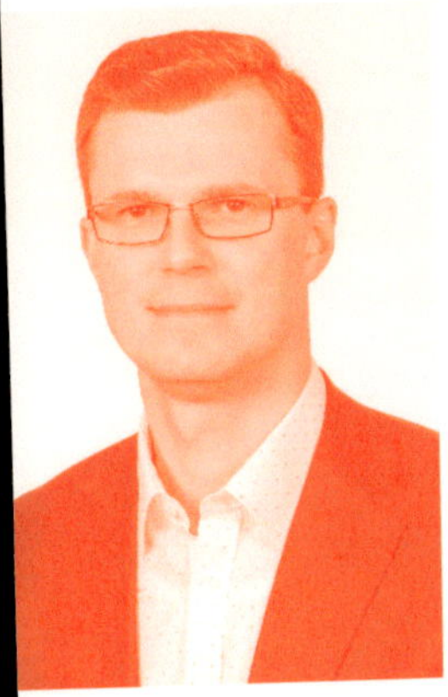
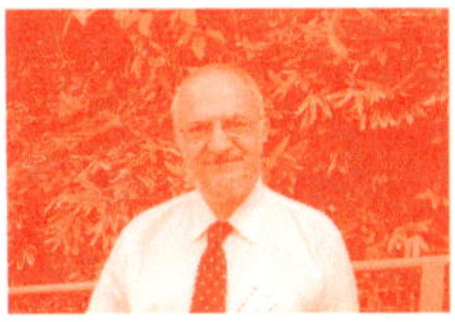
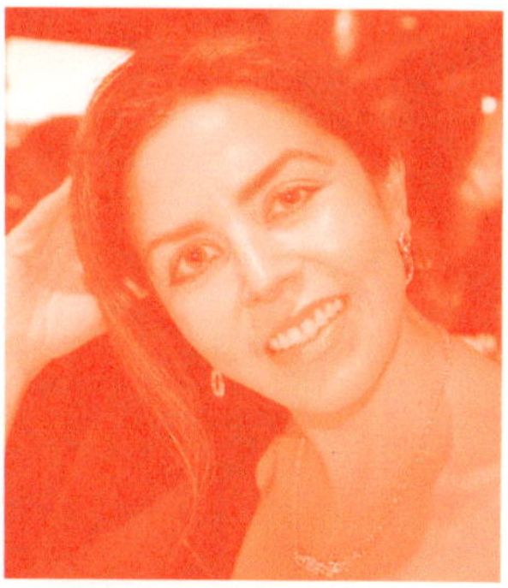

Supporting open minds since 2005

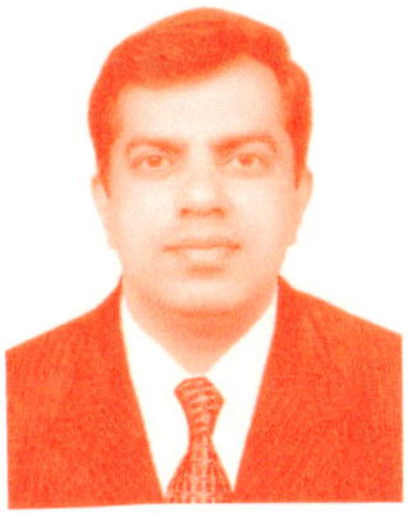
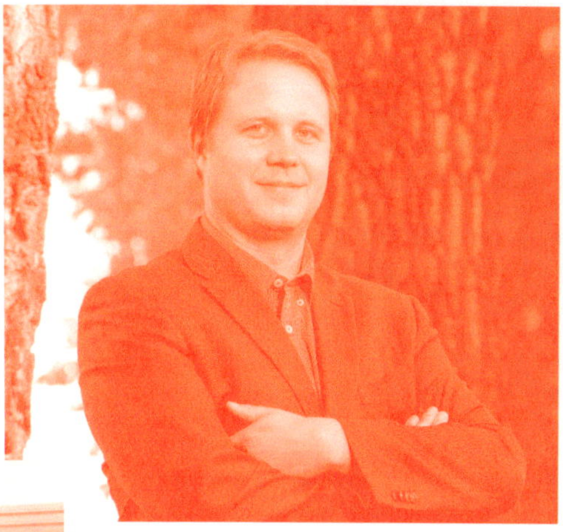
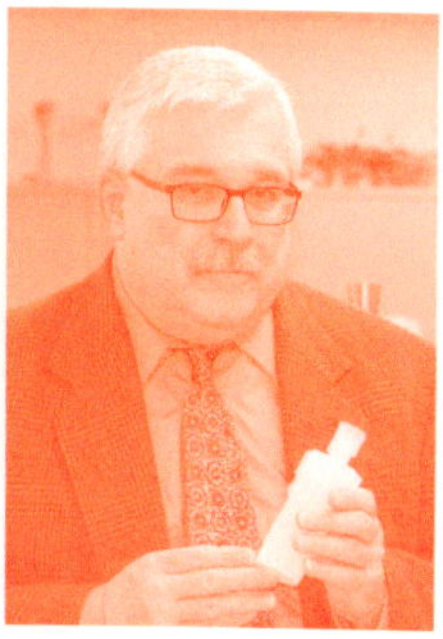
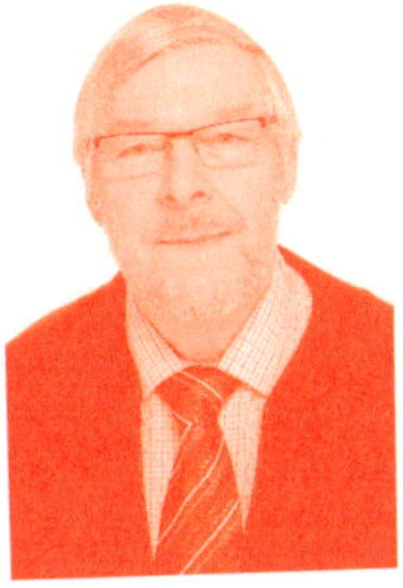
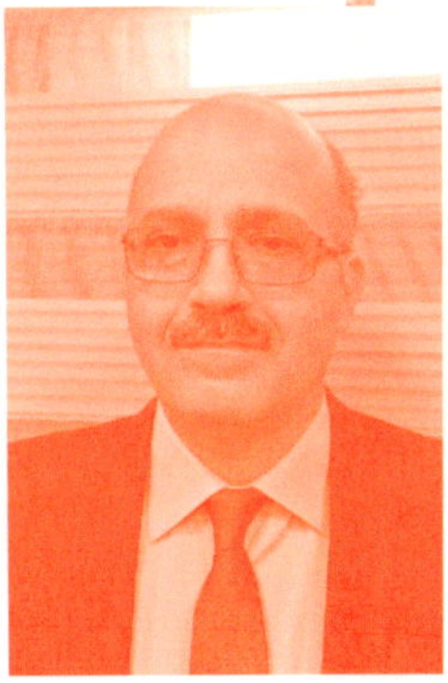
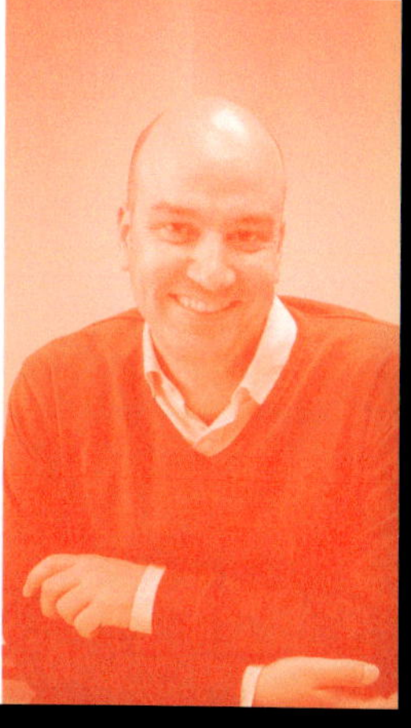
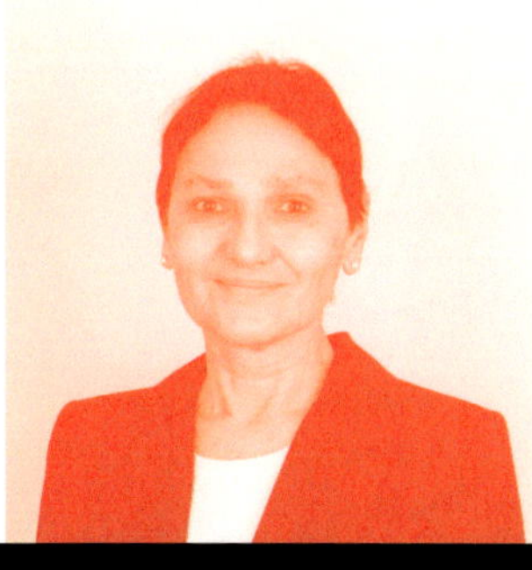

Different Areas of Physiotherapy
http://dx.doi.org/10.5772/intechopen.76695
Edited by Mintaze Kerem Gunel

Contributors
Marialuisa Gandolfi, Nicola Valè, Christian Geroin, Nicola Smania, Eleonora Dimitrova, Mirko Filippetti, Alessandro Picelli, Auwal Abdullahi, Shu Yan Ng, Mintaze Kerem Gunel

First published in London, United Kingdom, 2019 by IntechOpen
IntechOpen is the global imprint of INTECHOPEN LIMITED, registered in England and Wales, registration number: 11086078, The Shard, 25th floor, 32 London Bridge Street
London, SE19SG - United Kingdom
Printed in Croatia

British Library Cataloguing-in-Publication Data
A catalogue record for this book is available from the British Library

Additional hard and PDF copies can be obtained from orders@intechopen.com

Different Areas of Physiotherapy
Edited by Mintaze Kerem Gunel
p. cm.
Print ISBN 978-1-78985-589-0
Online ISBN 978-1-78985-590-6
eBook (PDF) ISBN 978-1-83880-323-0

Meet the editor

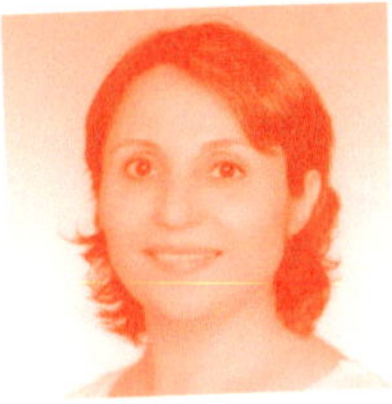

Dr. Mintaze Kerem Günel graduated from Hacettepe University, School of Physical Therapy and Rehabilitation, Turkey, in 1989. He earned a doctorate degree with his thesis, "Effectiveness of Johnstone Pressure Splints in Children with Spastic Cerebral Palsy." Since 1993, Dr. Günel has been clinically studying cerebral palsy. He works with the Children's Hospital at Hacettepe University, studying cerebral palsy in premature children. He is a member of the European Academy of Childhood Disability (EACD) and a national coordinator of Turkey. Dr. Günel currently works as a professor and the vice president of the Department of Physiotherapy and Rehabilitation, Hacettepe University.

Contents

Preface XI

Chapter 1 1
Introductory Chapter: Physiotherapy and Rehabilitation
by Mintaze Kerem Gunel, Cemil Ozal and Duygu Turker

Chapter 2 7
Movement Rehabilitation in Physiotherapy after Stroke: The Role of Constraint-Induced Movement Therapy
by Auwal Abdullahi

Chapter 3 27
Postural Control in Individuals with Parkinson's Disease
by Marialuisa Gandolfi, Nicola Valè, Mirko Filippetti, Eleonora Kirilova Dimitrova, Christian Geroin, Alessandro Picelli and Nicola Smania

Chapter 4 45
Physical Rehabilitation in the Management of Symptomatic Adult Scoliosis
by Shu-Yan Ng, Tsz-Ki Ho and Yin-Ling Ng

Preface

Different Areas of Physiotherapy provides comprehensive coverage of the key issues and perspectives in the field of physiotherapy. It presents the contemporary practice of physiotherapy with a focus on rehabilitation, including the nature of the body, the idea of independence, the rehabilitation process, and evidence-based and individual-centered practice. *Physiotherapy* encourages rehabilitation professionals to think about problem-solving and basic decision-making in a practice setting, presenting case studies to consolidate and apply learning.

Rehabilitation is a step-by-step process that helps people recover from injuries, trauma, health disorders, and more. The goal of rehabilitation is to help people function as effectively as possible after a life-changing event. Also, physiotherapy can be defined as a therapy method that focuses on the science of movement and helps people to restore, maintain, and maximize their physical strength, function, motion, and overall well-being by addressing underlying physical issues.

Physiotherapy encompasses rehabilitation, injury prevention, and health promotion and fitness. The profession employs a holistic approach to treatment, taking into account the patient's overall lifestyle.

This volume includes chapters written by experts from a wide range of clinical and academic backgrounds. Using a problem-solving approach, the book emphasizes the identification of symptoms in relation to impairment and disability rather than provides detailed descriptions of conditions related to physiotherapy. The authors use the current International Classification of Functioning, Disability and Health (ICF) to describe aspects of different posture and movement difficulties that an individual may experience. They provide guidance to help allied health professionals plan the appropriate therapy program for each patient and present the most frequently used and efficacious treatment methods.

The authors describe aspects related of ICF posture and movement difficulties which may occur as a result of some problems and gives guidance to help the allied health persons to plan the appropriate therapy program for each patient and all authors presented the most frequently used and treatment methods with efficacy and included references the end of each chapter.

Mintaze Kerem Gunel, PT, PhD.
Faculty of Health Sciences,
Department of Physiotherapy and Rehabilitation,
Turkey

Chapter 1

Introductory Chapter: Physiotherapy and Rehabilitation

Mintaze Kerem Gunel, Cemil Ozal and Duygu Turker

1. Introduction

Physiotherapy and rehabilitation have recently seen many practical innovations, evidences and major developments for specific interventions, not only in practical but also conceptual [1]. The approach to patients has moved from a predominantly medical biopsychosocial aspect and the need for organized specialist rehabilitation services has become equally important [2].

Physiotherapy is directed towards the movement necessities and potential of individuals, providing therapy and rehabilitation to enhance, maintain and restore maximum movement and functional skills throughout the lifespan [3]. Recent studies including systematic reviews and randomized controlled studies have emphasized proof for the clinical activity of physiotherapy interventions and rehabilitation for individuals with large different conditions range as orthopedic, neurologic, pulmonary, pediatric, rheumatologic or geriatric conditions [4].

The World Health Organization (WHO) describes rehabilitation as a process that supports individuals, experience or are under risk of functional limitation, to provide, enhance and maintain functionality in interaction with their environments' [5] and rehabilitation is based on way of thinking on problem-solving and fundamental decision-making in clinical interventions and apply learning. The problem-solving approach is based on description of symptoms in relation to structural and functional impairment and activity and participation limitation rather than only a specific description of different conditions related to physiotherapy.

"Physiotherapy and rehabilitation" are therapy process that are aimed to optimize functional and independence level and individual function limitations caused by pathologies which result in impairments. Rehabilitation is mainly focused the results of pathology rather than pathology itself. Physiotherapy and rehabilitation focus particularly on limitations which may affect physical functionality and activity and utilize a set of different interventions based on non-invasive and physical nature to assist progress toward functional objectives and aims [6]. Physiotherapy and rehabilitation are mostly focused on impairments related to mobility and functional or activity limitations as well as pain which are associated with musculoskeletal and neurological pathologies, injuries such as fractures and traumas, or cardio-pulmonary problems and treating them with exercises planned in line a target and manual mobilization approaches [7].

IntechOpen

2. International classification of functioning, disability and health (ICF) framework and physiotherapy and rehabilitation

Disablement models are a way of thinking about the results, impacts or sequelae of disease on functionality. Different classification schemes have been aimed to classify these sequelae. Recently, the WHO revised their scheme to produce ICF [6].

Disablement models are intended to show and create changes in perceptions of individuals with disabilities and meet their necessities to differentiate disease and pathology from the limitations they produced and these models were developed primarily for use by rehabilitation professionals. The expanded models try to have a more positive perspective on the changes caused by pathologies or disease and more intended for use by a wide range of people, including community, national and global institutions. The ICF has tried to change the perspective of disability from the native focus of outcomes of disease [6].

Within the ICF, physiotherapy and rehabilitation team can rely first on a worldwide accepted model providing a common language to describe and classify functionality, and the ICF is a framework for describing functioning and disability in relation to a health condition. It provides a common language and framework for documenting information on the functional changes after physiotherapy interventions [8].

3. ICF framework physiotherapy and rehabilitation interventions based on ICF

According to the ICF framework physiotherapy and rehabilitation approaches can be used according to these applications.

3.1 Approaches targeting impairments

The underlying assumption of these approaches is to prevent activity limitations by improving body functions and structures and different applications are described according to these aims.

Conventional methods for treatment of neuromusculoskeletal disorders primarily focus on the functioning of body structures, assuming that if joint play is restored and if stiff or contract muscles are relaxed and weak muscles strengthened, the ability to perform activities is automatically recovered [9].

3.2 Activity-oriented interventions

Activity-oriented movement strategies depend on activities rather than only impairments and aimed functionality with cognitive aspects, experience and intention that are fundamental for learning. An activity-oriented therapy program has a larger and much more prolonged positive effect than impairment-based structurally oriented therapy [10].

3.3 Environmental modification and assistive devices

Environmental adaptations can be used for different purposes. These objectives include increasing the functional independence of the child and reducing caregiver assistance [11]. Basic physiotherapy and rehabilitation interventions are listed in **Table 1**.

Physiotherapy and rehabilitation interventions	
Activity-based interventions	**Motor learning strategies**
Task-targeted training:	Strategy development
• Functional mobility skills	Feedback
• Daily living activities	Practice
Environmental context	Transfer of learning
Impairment oriented and augmented interventions	
Impairment interventions	**Augmented intervention**
Strength, power and endurance	Neuromuscular facilitations
Flexibility, range of motion and mobility	Proprioceptive neuromuscular facilitation
Coordination, agility and balance	Neurodevelopmental approaches
Gait and locomotion	Hands on mobilization techniques
Aerobic capacity/endurance	Neuromuscular electrical stimulation
Relaxation	Sensory stimulation
Compensatory interventions	
Substitution training	
• Alternate movement strategies	
• Less involved body segments	
Assistive/supportive devices	
Environmental modification	
Alternative daily life activities modification	

Table 1.
Physiotherapy and rehabilitation interventions [12].

4. Innovations in physiotherapy

Physiotherapy and rehabilitation are developed by using new approaches, activities and different new therapy models for different conditions, injuries, impairments and activity and participation limitations and assist people recover scope of mobility, and function as well as to maintain health condition in healthy individuals. It is important to think innovatively, and follow innovations to determine the best intervention for patient treatment. Innovations are mostly based on technological supported rehabilitation such as virtual reality games, rehabilitation robot or telerehabilitation [13].

5. Evidence-based physiotherapy

Evidence-based physiotherapy is an important and increasing issue in rehabilitation and physiotherapy. Although it is increasingly used worldwide, it is important to spread over among clinicians and researchers. Evidence-based practice has a significant movement of basic importance in delivery of healthcare worldwide [14].

Author details

Mintaze Kerem Gunel[1*], Cemil Ozal[1] and Duygu Turker[2]

1 Faculty of Physical Therapy and Rehabilitation, Hacettepe University, Ankara, Turkey

2 Department of Physiotherapy and Rehabilitation, Faculty of Gulhane Health Sciences, University of Health Sciences, Ankara, Turkey

*Address all correspondence to: mintaze@hacettepe.edu.tr

References

[1] Dannepfel P, Peolsson A, Nilsen P. What supports physiotherapists' use of research in clinical practice? A qualitative study in Sweden. Implementation Science. 2013;**8**:31

[2] Farre A, Rapley T. The new old (and old new) medical model: Four decades navigating the biomedical and psychosocial understandings of health and illness. Healthcare (Basel). 2017;**5**(4):88

[3] Stephensen D, Bladen M, Mclaughlin P. Recent advances in musculoskeletal physiotherapy for haemophilia. Therapeutic Advances in Hematology. 2018;**9**(8):227-237

[4] Howick J, Chalmers I, Glasziou P, et al. OCEBM Levels of Evidence Working Group. The Oxford 2011 Levels of Evidence. Oxford, UK: Oxford Centre for Evidence-Based Medicine; 2011

[5] World Health Organization (WHO), World Bank. World Report on Disability. Geneva: Author; 2011. Available from: https://www.who.int/disabilities/world_report/2011/en/ [Accessed: 14 May 2019]

[6] Cameron HM. Introduction. In: Cameron HM, Monroe GL, editors. Physical Rehabilitation for the Therapist Assistant. Saunders; 2011. pp. 1-8

[7] O'Sullivan SB, Schmitz TJ, Fulk GD. Physical Rehabilitation. Philadelphia: F.A. Davis Company; 2014

[8] Rauch A, Cıeza A, Stucki G. How to apply the international classification of functioning, disability and health (ICF) for rehabilitation management in clinical practice. European Journal of Physical and Rehabilitation Medicine. 2008;**44**:329-342

[9] Carlberg EB, Bower E. Manegement and treatment of postüral dysfunction in children with cerebral palsy. In: Hadders-Algra M, Carlber E, editors. Postural Control: A Key Issue in Developmental Disorders. London: MacKeith Press; 2008

[10] Mayston MJ. People with cerebral palsy: Effects and perspective of therapy. Neural Plasticity. 2001;**1-2**:51-69

[11] Ostensjo S, Brognen Carlberg E, Vollestad NK. The use and impact of assistive devices and other environmental modifications on everyday activities and care in young children with cerebral palsy. Disability and Rehabilitation. 2005;**27**:849-861

[12] Susan BO, Sullivan SB. Interventions to improve motor function. In: O'Sullivan SB, Schmitz JT, editors. Improving Functional Outcomes in Physical Rehabilitation. F.A. Davis Company; 2016. p. 2e

[13] Requejo PWC. Innovative technologies for rehabilitation and health promotion: What is the evidence? Physical Therapy. 2015;**95**(3):294-298

[14] Veras M, Kairy D, Paquet N. What is evidence-based physiotherapy. Physiotherapy Canada. 2016;**68**(2):95-96

Chapter 2

Movement Rehabilitation in Physiotherapy after Stroke: The Role of Constraint-Induced Movement Therapy

Auwal Abdullahi

Abstract

Stroke is increasingly becoming a global health problem. This is because it may lead to death, Long-term disability such as in motor function, and significant burden to the patients and their families. The disability can be prevented or rehabilitated using a physiotherapy technique known as constraint-induced movement therapy (CIMT). The CIMT comprises of task practice with the affected limb, constraint of the unaffected limb, and transfer package to foster compliance and increase the amount of task repetition. It helps to reestablish normal motor control through facilitating changes in physiological functions of the brain, improvement in real-world arm use, and movement precision and quality. However, its protocols vary. Some protocols use number of hours and others use number of repetitions to determine the intensity or the amount of task practice. This chapter argued that CIMT is effective, but the protocols that use a number of hours of task practice are not clear and are resource intensive; and as such they could interfere with the process of clinical decision making. Consequently, it proposed the use of a number of repetitions of task practice to determine the intensity or the amount of task practice and extending the application of CIMT to those with severe impairments after stroke.

Keywords: stroke, motor recovery, neuroscience, constraint-induced movement therapy, rehabilitation

1. Introduction

This chapter reviews the roles played by constraint-induced movement therapy (CIMT) in the rehabilitation of movement impairment following stroke. The chapter discusses these issue under three major sections and a conclusion section. The sections are overview on stroke, control of human movement, and the role of CIMT. The section on overview on stroke comprises of definition of stroke, etiology of stroke, pathophysiology of stroke, epidemiology of stroke, and consequences of stroke. The section on control of human movement consists only of nervous system control of movement in health and disease. The section on the role of CIMT consists of constraint-induced movement therapy: historical background and neuroscientific basis, components of CIMT, protocols of constraint-induced movement therapy, effects of constraint-induced movement therapy, and constraint-induced movement therapy: the future perspective. Information from all the sections to be discussed is needed by the physiotherapist in order to be able to make an effective clinical decision during application of CIMT in people with stroke.

2. Overview on stroke

2.1 Definition

World over, stroke has become a major public health issue. It is defined as "a rapidly developing clinical signs of focal (or global) disturbance of cerebral function, lasting more than 24 h or leading to death, with no apparent cause other than that of vascular origin" [1]. This definition seems outdated since presently there are advances in prevention, diagnosis, and management of stroke, which led to so many people surviving stroke and living with long-term disabilities. Additionally, stroke is a compendium of neurovascular syndromes with diverse presentations, and the 24 h time limit is not sacrosanct as minutes or few hours of stroke event can lead to severe and/or permanent damage [2]. Consequently, attempts were made to reassess the definition of transient ischemic attack and stroke [2, 3]. A high-powered committee of experts deliberated and defined the conditions; thus, stroke is classically characterized as a neurological deficit attributed to an acute focal injury of the central nervous system (CNS) by a vascular cause, including cerebral infarction, intracerebral hemorrhage (ICH), and subarachnoid hemorrhage (SAH), and is a major cause of disability and death worldwide [2]. This definition included the vascular causes of the condition. Thus, from the foregoing, it can be seen that stroke results from various vascular events and can manifest as varied forms of neurological signs and symptoms.

2.2 Etiology

As stated in the definitions by Hatano and Sacco and his colleagues, the causes of stroke are of vascular origins [1, 2]. These sources are ischemia and intracerebral and subarachnoid hemorrhage, which may cause cerebral infarction. Ischemia simply means reduction in blood supply to brain cells, which could be due to occlusion as a result of the presence of either thrombus (a blood clot) or embolus (a moving blood clot) or stenosis (narrowing or reduction in the caliber of the arteries) [4]. The embolus usually may originate from the arteries or the heart as a result of conditions such as atrial fibrillation, sinoatrial disorder, recent acute myocardial infarction (AMI), marantic or subacute bacterial endocarditis, cardiac tumors, and valvular disorders, both native and artificial [5]. The intracerebral hemorrhage (ICH) and subarachnoid hemorrhage (SAH), which mean rupture or leakage of the tiny or very small blood vessels in the brain, are mainly caused by the elevated or increased intracranial pressure and sustained weakening of walls of blood vessels usually as a result of a long-standing high blood pressure [6]. Although majority of stroke cases are due to ischemia, in very rare cases, hemorrhagic and ischemic stroke can occur concurrently [7]. However, when stroke occurred as either ischemic or hemorrhagic, the latter usually leads to poor prognosis including mortality than ischemic stroke [8].

2.3 Pathophysiology

The human brain under normal circumstances receives 20% of the cardiac output [9]. This output is responsible for cerebral blood flow (CBF) whose normal value in adults is about 50–55 ml/100 g/min. This makes the brain tissues to be rich and abundant in oxygen and glucose necessary for major metabolic processes at all times.

Thus, damage to the brain tissues due to reduced blood flow depends on the extent of the reduction to the tissues and probably for how long the reduction persists. If the CBF reduced to about 14 ± 2 ml/100 g/min, the damage is usually reversible, and the affected area is known as ischemic penumbra. The penumbra is a region of functionally impaired, but structurally intact, tissues. Thus, this area of penumbra is the one that offers hope for recovery in case of therapy and rehabilitation. On the other hand, if the CBF reduced to about 6 ml/100 g/min, the damage is usually irreversible, and the affected area is known as the core. The core is the region of infarction. This is because the human brain is not endowed with respiratory reserve; it has low capacity for oxygen reserve, and this makes it to heavily depend on aerobic respiration. Any event that will alter its circulatory process and interfere with the aerobic respiration can cause damage to the brain cells. However, the abundant collateral circulation in the brain ensures that the effect of the damage is limited to some parts of the brain.

The events that bring about the alteration or impairment in blood circulation in the brain come in two ways: ischemia and hemorrhage. Ischemia is usually in the form of thrombosis in large and small vessels, embolism with or without cardiac and/or arterial factor, systematic hypoperfusion, and venous thrombosis. The mechanism of brain cell damage due to ischemia is through depletion of oxygen and glucose with attendant reduced capacity to produce energy-releasing compounds such as the adenosine triphosphate (ATP) [10]. The molecule ATP is important for cellular metabolic processes. This creates a vicious cycle of lack of essential molecules such as oxygen and glucose for the survival of the cells and eventually causes cellular death. The extent of the damage is, however, a factor of the location, severity, and the duration of ischemia. That is to say, the longer the duration of the ischemia, the more extensive the damage will be.

The mechanisms of cellular death due to ischemia often come in many ways. One of these ways comes through the damage or dysfunction of the mitochondria. The mitochondria are the energy storage or power house of the cells [11]. Dysfunction or damage of the mitochondria will result in depletion of energy required to initiate and sustain physiologic processes such as the normal function of ion gradient, which results in ionic imbalance. The ionic imbalance pertains to the loss of potassium in exchange of sodium, chloride, and calcium ions [12]. This ionic imbalance leads to intracellular accumulation of fluid, which manifests as swelling of neuronal cells and glia that will eventually lead to the death of these cells. Another way in which neuronal cell death can occur due to ischemia is through excessive release of excitatory neurotransmitters such as the glutamate and aspartate. These neurotransmitters release will further complicate the damage to the brain cells. Other ways through which cellular death occur include production of oxygen-free radicals and reactive oxygen species (ROS), and apoptosis. Free radicals and the ROS react with a number of cellular and extracellular elements including the vascular endothelium and cause cell death. Apoptosis occurs in response to release of proapoptotic molecules such as cytochrome c and apoptosis-inducing factor from mitochondria due to gene expression of Bcl-2 and p53.

The whole process resembles blocking the water supply to a flower. If the blockage continues, the flower begins to shrink gradually and eventually dies off. Thus, whatever the pathophysiologic process that takes place, the result is that ischemia or reperfusion causes cell death, and this in turn causes impairment in brain functions [13]. The pathophysiologic process of stroke is simplified in **Figure 1**.

2.4 Epidemiology of stroke

Many people around the world suffer stroke. According to the World Heart Federation, annually about 15 million people suffer stroke, out of which about 40% die and 33.33% live with long-term disability [14]. This shows that about 60%

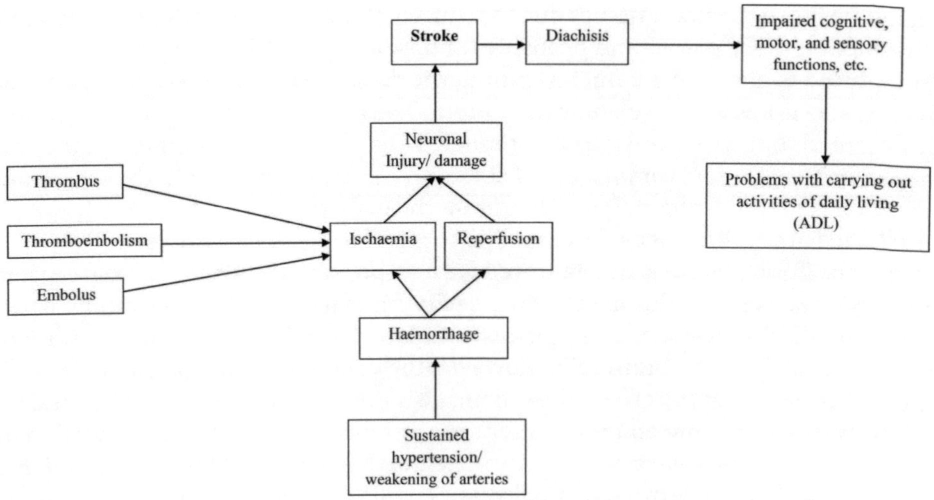

Figure 1.
Schematic representation of pathophysiology of stroke and its consequences.

survives stroke probably due to improved stroke management over the last few decades. Equally, the percentage of those who live with long-term disability also calls for public health concern. Thus, improving rehabilitation services for stroke survivors is much needed. However, the incidence of stroke seems to vary between different regions of the world. In many developed countries, the incidence of stroke is declining even though the actual number of strokes is increasing because of the aging population [14, 15]. In contrast, in the developing countries, the incidence of stroke is increasing. For example, about 1.3 million people suffer stroke every year with about 75% surviving it, and the incidence is predicted to increase with high incidence of death in Latin America, the Middle East, and sub-Saharan Africa in a few decades to come probably due to lack of standard care for stroke [14].

Many factors can put one at the risk of developing stroke. The risk factors for stroke can be divided into modifiable and nonmodifiable ones. The modifiable risk factors include high blood pressure, heart disease, hypercholesterolemia, physical inactivity, smoking, alcohol consumption, diabetes mellitus, psychosocial stress and depression, and kidney diseases [16]. The nonmodifiable risk factors include gender, race, and genetic factors. For gender as a nonmodifiable risk factor, there are varied reports on whether stroke occurs more in women or men and vice versa, though they are mostly in favor of high incidence in women. According to a study by Petrea and colleagues, stroke occurs more in women than men, though there is no significant difference between men and women in terms of stroke severity, subtype, and case fatality [17]. These variations may probably represent the social structure of a given population. Consequently, the incidence between men and women may be because of one gender reporting to the clinic more than the other in a given population. Secondly, the distribution of gender in the population can also play a role. In addition to all that was mentioned, women tend to have poorer functional outcomes following stroke [18]. Furthermore, whatever the cause of a stroke, its incidence imposes a huge financial burden on patients and their families and can cost governments millions of dollars as direct and indirect costs depending on the country and the particular healthcare system.

2.5 Consequences of stroke

Stroke results in impairment of brain functions, cognitive, motor, and sensory/perceptual functions [13]. Examples of these impairments include decreased movement quality, impaired movement coordination, gait and balance problems, vascular dementia, memory impairment, emotional disturbances, and hemispatial neglect. The motor impairment is significant since movement is important for humans' daily functioning. The consequences of impairment of brain functions following stroke include difficulty in carrying out activities of daily living such as washing, dressing, bathing and difficulty in carrying out previously enjoyed leisure activities [19]. Normal functions of the brain are required in our daily life activities and participation. Therefore, rehabilitation is important to help patient recover or live an independent life as much as possible. In physiotherapy practice, CIMT is used for the rehabilitation of movement impairment after stroke.

3. Nervous system control of movement in health and disease

One of the major functions of the nervous system is the control of human movement, which is essential for our daily functioning and participation. This control occurs in top-down, bottom-up, and parallel manner using different parts of the central nervous system. The CNS structures responsible for the control of human movement include the cerebral cortex, basal ganglia, brainstem, cerebellum, and thalamus that are contained in the diencephalon and spinal cord, which are complemented by the peripheral feedback [20, 21]. The functions of these various structures are summarized in **Figure 2**.

The cerebral cortex functions for cognition, perception, and behavior. The cerebral cortex integrates these aforementioned functions to help execute human movements. It consists mainly of three important structures that are closely related with each other, the motor cortex, the premotor area, and the primary motor area. The main function of the motor cortex is sending inputs/commands through the corticospinal tract and corticobulbar system to the brainstem and the spinal cord [20]. The premotor area functions alongside other parts of the brain in movement

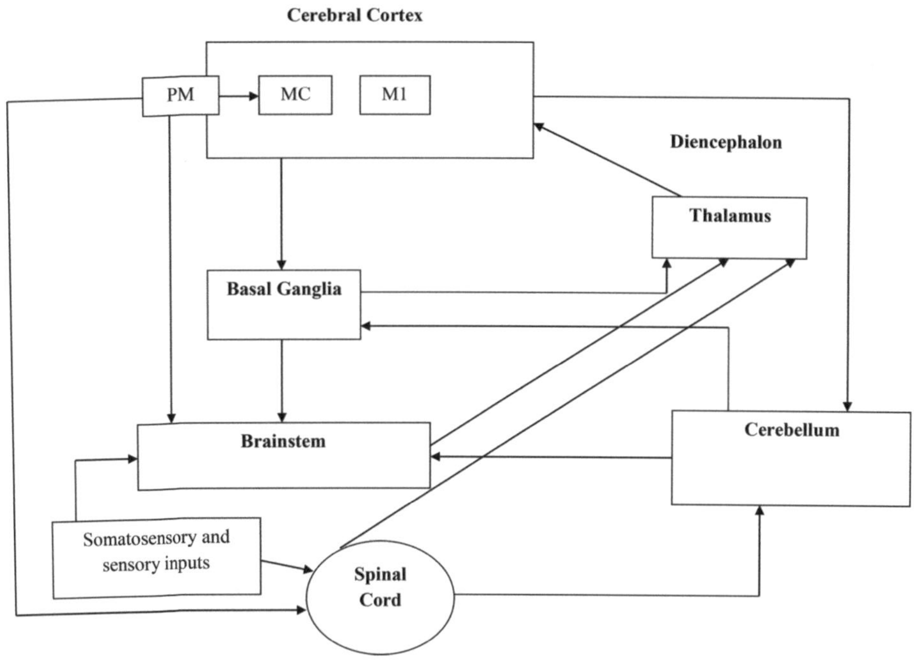

Figure 2.
Schematic representation of nervous control of human movement. PM, premotor cortex; MC, motor cortex; M1, primary motor cortex.

programming, selection of what to do, and identification of objects in space [20, 22]. It sends most of its outputs directly to the motor cortex, and some to the brainstem and the spinal cord [23]. The basal ganglia are a collection of nuclei at the base of the brain that are involved in higher-order cognitive functions like planning the strategies of movement [24]. These nuclei receive inputs from most parts of the cerebral cortex and send back their outputs to the motor cortex by the way of the thalamus.

The brainstem is important for the control of posture and locomotion. Postural control is essential for proper execution of movement. This is possible due to the presence of important nuclei in the brainstem, which include vestibular nuclei, red nuclei, and reticular nuclei [20, 21]. The brainstem receives somatosensory inputs from the skin and muscles of the head and sensory inputs from the vestibular and visual systems. Similarly, nuclei in the brainstem control outputs to the neck, face, and eyes. The cerebellum receives inputs from the spinal cord and the cerebral cortex detailing about movement and planning of movement, respectively. In addition, it sends output to the brainstem. The main functions of the cerebellum are comparing the intended movement with sensory signals and update the movement commands when the movement goes abnormally. Secondly, it helps in modulating range and force of movements. The thalamus is contained in the diencephalon, and most of the outputs from the basal ganglia, the spinal cord, the brainstem, and the cerebellum are processed via it. The spinal cord is at the lower level of the movement control hierarchy. It receives somatosensory information from the muscles, joints, and skin and sends information to the higher centers. However, following stroke, the functions of these various structures of the brain become impaired in such a way that movement is no longer well planned, coordinated, modulated, and integrated. The aim of rehabilitation is to reestablish these various integrated functions for normal movement control. Consequently, constraint-induced movement therapy (CIMT) is used to reestablish the normal nervous control of human movement.

4. Role of constraint in movement rehabilitation after stroke

4.1 Constraint-induced movement therapy: historical background and neuroscientific basis

Movement is important in every human's endeavors; it is essential for the performance of most of our daily activities. However, after a stroke, our ability to move may be impaired. This is due to the impairment in normal movement control as a result of damage to some areas of the brain. To help reestablish normal movement control following stroke, constraint-induced movement therapy is used [25, 26]. Constraint-induced movement therapy (CIMT) is a movement rehabilitation technique, which aims to counteract learned nonuse acquired after stroke [26, 27]. The learned nonuse phenomenon is an acquired behavior exhibited by patients following stroke that makes them not to use the affected limb in functional activities. It is said to be due to failure to carry out tasks after unsuccessful attempts as a result of depression of functions of the central nervous system, pain or fatigue following the injury. This acquired behavior may set off a vicious cycle of impairments comprising of decreased movement, decreased cortical representation of the affected part of the body, and compensatory behavior that may also decrease use of the affected part [28]. The mechanisms of learned nonuse phenomenon are depicted in **Figure 3**. Please refer to the articles by Taub and his colleagues for more details on the learned nonuse [27, 28]. Although, the description of the learned nonuse phenomenon by Taub has been challenged, modified, and expanded to include psychosocial and structural factors that can lead to the acquired behavior [29], his explanation has provided researchers

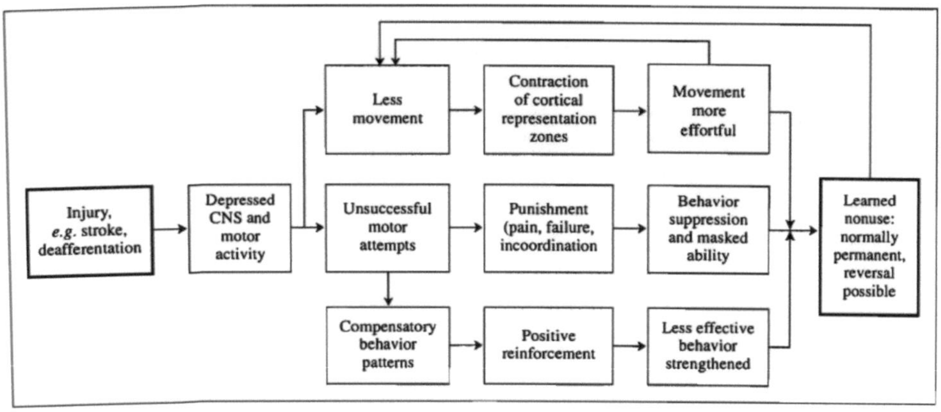

Figure 3.
The learned nonuse phenomenon (reproduced with permission from Edward Taub).

and clinicians with the foundation for designing restorative rehabilitation techniques enabling people with stroke regain functions. The examples of these techniques have been seen in forced use and CIMT.

The origin of CIMT has been credited to the work of Edward Taub, though he acknowledged previous researchers' contribution to the understanding of this phenomenon [25]. Here, monkeys received surgical abolition of somatic sensation of one or the two forelimbs. Thereafter, they were trained based on some learning principles. The abolition of somatic sensation conditioned the monkeys to never use the limbs again. However, the animals were forced to use the affected limb as soon as the unaffected limb is constrained. Additionally, it was noted that the use of the affected limb was further strengthened when the animal was rewarded with food after a successful attempt. The use of the limb was achieved through breaking task into manageable components in a process known as shaping. Subsequently, this protocol was first translated to a patient with chronic stroke in which his unaffected upper limb was constrained for about 90% of the waking hours and patients with chronic stroke and brain injury [26, 30]. This variant of CIMT is known as forced use. The current and widely used variant of CIMT was started on chronic patients who received constraint of the unaffected limb for 90% of the waking hours and task practice with the affected limb for 6 h for 10 days [27]. So far, there are many variants of CIMT in forms of randomized controlled trials (RCT), single case experimental studies, case reports, and so forth. In fact, as of now, there are not less than 500 studies of CIMT including a highly rigorous multicenter RCT known as the EXCITE trial [31].

In addition to the explanations above, thus far CIMT has been extended to the rehabilitation of many conditions such as cerebral palsy, brachial plexus injury, spinal cord injury, multiple sclerosis, aphasia, and hearing impairments [32–36]. All these reported improvement in the outcomes of interest. Furthermore, currently CIMT is used for both upper and lower limbs [37, 38]. However, the studies in lower limbs are still few, and therefore, more studies need to be carried out to determine the effect of CIMT in lower limb motor impairment after stroke. This will help in translating the opportunities gained with upper limb CIMT and possibly further researchers' understanding of the mechanisms of recovery of motor function following stroke.

4.2 Components of constraint-induced movement therapy

The basic components of CIMT include repetitive task/shaping practice with the affected limb, constraint of the unaffected limb, and transfer package [39]. Task practice involves carrying out the usual everyday tasks or activities such as brushing, cooking, washing plates, playing tennis, kicking or throwing a ball, and picking up a cup and taking it to the mouth to drink from it [40, 41]. In shaping practice, similar tasks as in task practice are carried out; however, they are broken down into manageable components in which the participant will have to master a component before proceeding to another [40–42]. For example, when a participant is to learn how to pick up a cup and take it to the mouth to drink from it, he will be taught to learn how to grasp the cup, then pick it up, and the rest follows. Constraining the unaffected limb involves use of slings, mitts, or any possibly practicable orthotic device to prevent the use of the limb [42]. Sometimes, this can be achieved through conscious restriction of the use of the unaffected limb by the patient. The transfer package is any method used to foster compliance with task/shaping practice and the constraint components of CIMT [41]. The methods used include the use of logbook, diary, everyday administration of motor activity log, monitoring by caregivers, and practice outside the laboratory (e.g., at home).

In the literature, importance of repetitive task/shaping practice in being an essential component responsible for improvement following CIMT has been underscored. However, according to Taub and colleagues, transfer package is very key to improvement in function following CIMT [43]. This finding probably confirms the importance of task or shaping repetition as transfer package is meant to foster compliance and use of the affected limb outside laboratory. In essence, transfer package helps to achieve more repetition. Similarly, constraint ensures that use of the constrained limb is restricted, while the use of the affected limb is maximized. This is also akin to encouraging more repetitions with the affected limb. Pooling all these arguments together, we can see that the other components of CIMT, constraint, and transfer package work to provide high repetition of task or shaping practice. This is more especially that it has been reported for the upper limbs that there was no significant difference whether constraint is used or not during CIMT [44]. However, studies on CIMT for the lower limb need to determine whether use of constraint is necessary, tolerable, or even practicable. Some studies on upper limb have indicated some compliance or tolerability of the participants with constraint [45, 46].

4.3 Protocols of constraint-induced movement therapy

Constraint-induced movement therapy has evolved over the years to have many different protocols. The protocols involve either modification of the task/shaping practice, constraint or both components of CIMT; or even the process or setting of its administration. These protocols include using hours as measure of intensity of task/shaping practice, using number of repetitions as measure of intensity of task/shaping practice, home-based CIMT, use of automated constraint-induced therapy extension (AutoCITE), and CIMT without constraint [38, 47–50]. See **Table 1** for the details of these different protocols. The protocol that uses number of repetitions is relatively a new approach. Therefore, its details are represented in **Table 2**.

One of the concerns about the standard CIMT is the issue of compliance since it seems to have a long duration of tasks/shaping practice of 6 h or less [51]. However, studies such as those by Kaplon and his colleagues and Stock and his colleagues have all indicated that the time spent practicing task/shaping fell short of what is being claimed [52, 53]. Additionally, many studies have shown that the shorter duration CIMT, the protocol that uses less than or 3 h of task/shaping practice, provides better outcomes [54, 55]. In contrast, the protocol using number of repetition has been touted to be feasible, easier, and may provide better compliance and complements the transfer package component as it takes on the elements of self-management [45, 56]. Recently, it has been shown to be as effective as the one using number of hours [48, 49]. Furthermore, a virtual reality-amplified arm training of just 30 minutes

Protocol	Task/shaping practice	Constraint	Transfer package
Use of hours	Practice for 0.5–6 h for ≥ 10 days	Constraint for 2 h or more or for 90% of the waking hours	Logbook, diary, everyday administration of motor activity log, monitoring by caregivers, practicing at home, etc.
Without constraint	Same as above	No any constraint	Same as above
Home-based CIMT	Same as above, but practice is done at home	Same as above	Same as above
Use of AutoCITE	Same as in use of hours, but practice is administered through the use of a computerized mechanical system	Same as above	Same as above
Use of number of repetitions	300–600 repetitions in two or three sessions per day	Constraint for 90% of the waking hours	Same as above

Table 1.
Different protocols of CIMT.

proved very effective at improving motor outcomes at 6 weeks postintervention and 3 months follow-up [57]. This technique known as reinforcement-induced therapy uses virtual reality system with the sole aim of optimizing proper practice with the affected arm during rehabilitation. Similarly, an automated delivery of CIMT has been used [51]. This form of delivery of CIMT is aimed at fostering compliance with the CIMT protocol. Therefore, the goal of future CIMT protocols should be aimed at improving compliance in order to achieve the massed practice of the technique. This type of protocol as reported in some previous studies can be administered in the form of a distributed practice [48, 58]. A distributed practice is a type of practice in which the practice is divided into sessions per day [42]. Probably, distributed practice will help do away with overwhelm; fatigue and possibly anxiety patients may have and help encourage them perform the required intensity of practice per day.

4.4 Effects of constraint-induced movement therapy

Effectiveness of a given rehabilitation intervention can be said to be sound if it is evaluated on different outcomes. This will enable the intervention to have a strong theoretical basis. For CIMT, its effects have been investigated on impairments such as

Tasks	No. of repetitions per session	No. of sessions per day	No. of days per week	No. of weeks
(1) Writing the letter A	20	2 or 3	5 or 7	2 or more
(2) Picking up a cup, taking it to the mouth, and drinking from it	20	2 or 3	5 or 7	2 or more
(3) Drawing a circle	20	2 or 3	5 or 7	2 or more
(4) Transferring an object from one place to another on a table	20	2 or 3	5 or 7	2 or more
(5) Imitation of teeth brushing with the middle or the index finger	20	2 or 3	5 or 7	2 or more

Table 2.
Example of the protocols of tasks/shaping practice for the CIMT using number of repetitions.

neurophysiological and behavioral, real-world arm use, motor function, activities of daily living, quality of life, and kinematics [31, 55, 59–64]. Recently, it has been demonstrated that neurophysiological changes following CIMT well correlate with motor function [48, 64]. The examples of effects of CIMT and the effects based on the International Classification of Functioning, Disability and Health (ICF) model are summarized in **Table 3** and **Figure 4**, respectively. These effects are measured using outcome measures such as Wolf motor function test (WMFT), action research arm test (ARAT), nine peg hole test (NPHT), motor activity log (MAL), motor function subscale of Fugl-Meyer assessment (FM), upper limb self-efficacy test (UPSET), functional magnetic resonance imaging (fMRI), and transmagnetic stimulation (TMS) [27, 30, 65–72]. The WMFT, the ARAT, the FM, and the JPHT are measures of motor function [30, 68, 69, 73]. The fMRI and TMS are measures of neurophysiological functions [70, 72]. The MAL is a measure of real-world arm use [27, 70, 71]. The UPSET is a measure of confidence in the use of the upper limb after stroke [67]. However, the effects are restricted to only those who have mild to moderate impairment. Consequently, the inclusion criteria used during CIMT include patients who have 10° and 30° of interphalangeal and wrist joints extension, respectively, or those that have some level of motor activity enough to enable them practice some tasks with the limb [40, 59, 73]. Thus, the existing protocol of CIMT is not a one size fits all kind of rehabilitation technique, though the need to investigate how its application can be extended to all forms of degree or level of impairment arises.

Effects	Examples
Neurophysiological effects	Increase in gray matter, increase in cortical map, increase in cortical activation, decreased transcallosal inhibition, improvement in central conduction time, improvement in resting motor threshold, and prolongation of cortical silent period
Kinematics	Efficient temporal and spatial movements, improved preplanned movement and control
Behavioral	Improved real-world arm use, improved use of the hand in activities requiring fine motor control, improved motor function, improved gait and balance

Table 3.
Effects of constraint-induced movement therapy (CIMT).

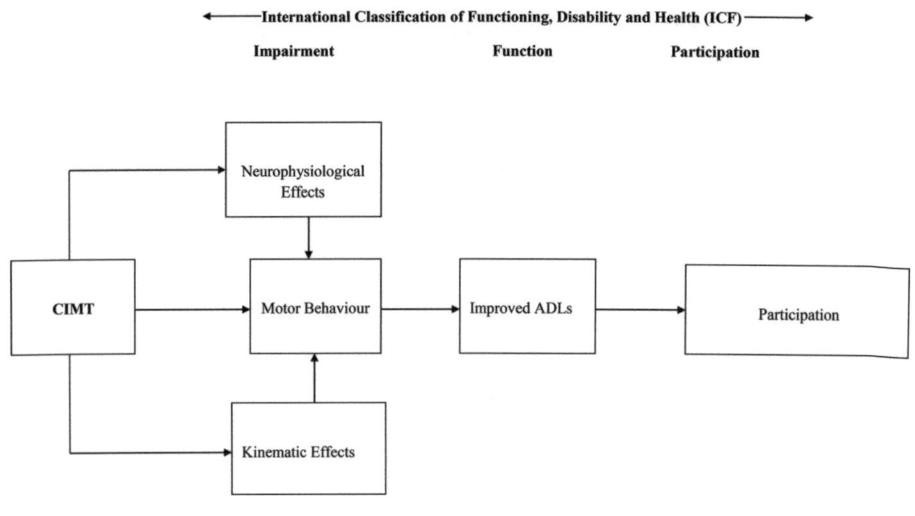

Figure 4.
Schematic representation of the effects of constraint-induced movement therapy (CIMT) in stroke patients. ADL, activities of daily living.

4.5 Constraint-induced movement therapy: the future perspective

At the moment, CIMT is administered only to the patients who have mild to moderate impairment. These are those who can to some extent perform some motor activity with the affected part. However, it is possible to integrate mental practice and motor imagery in the existing protocols of CIMT for the benefits of those with severe impairment bearing in mind the neurophysiological effect of CIMT and its relationship with motor function [64], and the role of mirror neurons when actions of a second or third person are observed or when task performance is imagined [74]. This perspective is for the benefit of those who may have severe impairment—those who do not have any appreciable motor activity enough to enable them perform any task. These forms of CIMT may be called passive CIMT (pCIMT) and imagery CIMT (iCIMT), respectively. For the pCIMT, the task/shaping practice should be carried out in high repetition with the affected limb similar to the repetition in the standard CIMT, and the unaffected limb should be constrained for 90% of the waking hours or less depending on the therapist's clinical decision. However, the transfer package component may be initiated or deferred until the patients improve in their motor ability that they can use to practice. This too depends on the therapist's clinical decision and reasoning. Similarly, for the iCIMT, the patient should be made to observe a second person or third person performing task/shaping practice to the required number of repetition as in the normal CIMT protocol. Here, the unaffected limb may or may not be constrained.

Another possible perspective is to use the number of repetition as a measure of intensity of task/shaping practice during CIMT. Already, there are indications that these types of protocols seem to be easier and have similar effectiveness compared to the one using number of hours [48, 49]. This is because number of repetition of task is important for motor recovery [45, 51, 58].

4.6 A hypothetical case to help enhance problem solving, clinical decision making, and clinical reasoning in constraint-induced movement therapy

Mr. MM is a 67-year-old community dwelling man who had a stroke 10 days earlier. Before his stroke, he was a very active subsistent farmer. He woke up the morning he had the stroke and realized that he was unable to move any part of his body. Upon realizing his condition, his family rushed him to a nearby secondary health facility where he was diagnosed with a stroke and started receiving care accordingly. According to clinical assessments and reports, he had ischemic stroke involving the left hemisphere. Mr. MM's main presentations were inability to sit or stand and walk without help from the formal or informal caregivers, and inability to use his right upper limb for any activity. Other presentations include inability to maintain his position in sitting without help.

In order to design a rehabilitation program using CIMT say for the upper limb for this patient, we need to first of all identify his problems. We can identify his problem by assessing his level of activity with the upper limb using, for example, Wolf motor function test or motor activity log, and being aware of the degree of freedom at the joints of the upper limb [27, 31]. Similarly, we can assess the range of motion (ROM) in the individual joints and assess the limb for spasticity, for instance, using modified Ashworth scale (MAS) [75]. Thereafter, we can develop alternative protocols of CIMT for him. For instance, we can decide to plan 6 h or less of task/shaping practice for the right limb with constraint for 90% or less of the waking hours, or we can plan for 300 or more of task/shaping practice for the right limb with constraint for 90% or less of the waking hours divided into two or more sessions per day. Additionally, we may decide to manage the patient at home, in the clinic, or provide him with the skills to self-manage. In particular, self-management is important for positive outcomes after stroke [76, 77].

After making an informed clinical decision on the choice of the best alternative or protocol, we can then administer it and reassess or monitor and evaluate its progress after sometime. If it works fine, we can decide to continue with it; if it does not provide any appreciable outcome, we can decide to choose another alternative protocol. This is the clinical reasoning. However, the existing studies on CIMT do not especially emphasize on clinical reasoning, rather they give a straightjacket prescription of what should be done throughout the period of care whether the patients improve better or not. Clinical reasoning is important to physiotherapy practice [78]. The process of problem solving, clinical decision making, and clinical reasoning in constraint-induced movement therapy is represented in **Figure 5**.

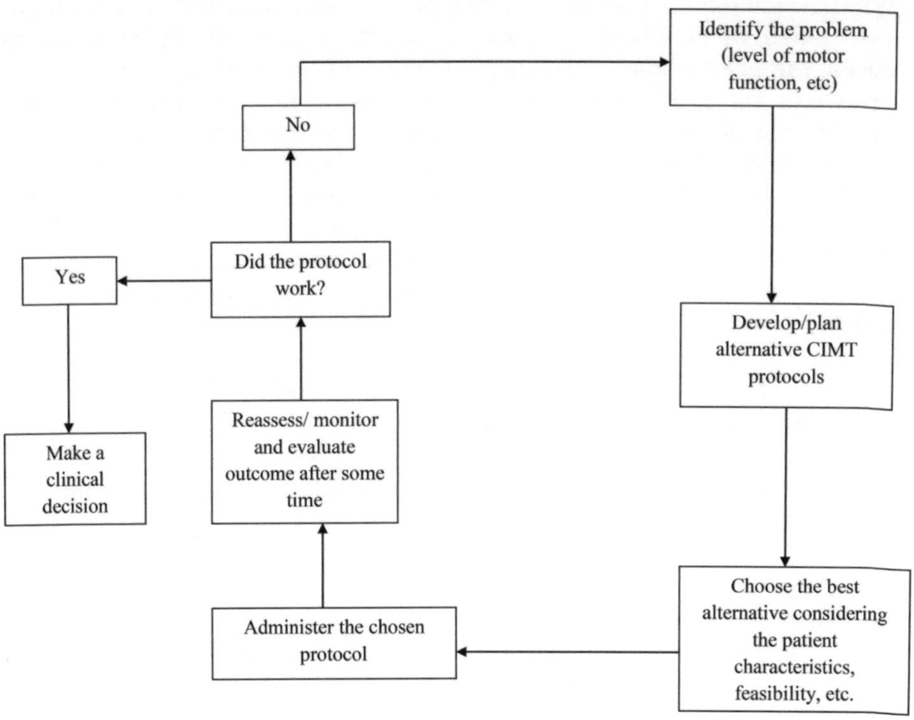

Figure 5.
Problem solving, clinical decision making, and clinical reasoning in CIMT.

5. Conclusion

Constraint-induced movement therapy (CIMT) plays a major role in the rehabilitation of movement after stroke. Its effects range from improved real-world use of the arm, motor function, neurophysiological functions, kinematics, and quality of life. The problem is that CIMT is not done for all categories of patients with stroke. It is done for only those with mild to moderate impairment. Additionally, there are varied protocols of CIMT. Some protocols use number of hours and some others use number of repetitions of tasks/shaping practice. The protocols that use number of hours of task practice are not clear and are resource intensive, and as such, they could interfere with the process of clinical decision making. Consequently, the use of number of repetitions of task practice to determine the intensity or the amount of task practice may be more appropriate. Secondly, there is a need to extend the use of

CIMT application to those patients with severe impairments after stroke probably by asking the patients to wear constraint on the unaffected limb and imagine they are practicing tasks with the affected limb. However, skills in problem solving, clinical decision making, and clinical reasoning are required by the physiotherapist in order to make an effective use of CIMT. These skills may be acquired through reflective practice and continuing professional development.

Conflict of interest declaration

The author does not have any conflict of interest to declare.

Author details

Auwal Abdullahi
Department of Physiotherapy, Faculty of Health Sciences, Bayero University Kano, Nigeria

*Address all correspondence to: aabdullahi.pth@buk.edu.ng

References

[1] Hatano S. Experience from a multicentre stroke register: A preliminary report. Bullettin of the World Health Organisation. 1976;**54**(5):541-553

[2] Sacco RL, Kasner SE, Broderick JP, Caplan LR, Connors JJ, Culebras A, et al. An updated definition of stroke for the 21st century: A statement for healthcare professionals from the American Heart Association/ American Stroke Association. Stroke. 2013;**44**(7):2064-2089. DOI: 10.1161/ STR.0b013e318296aeca

[3] Easton JD, Saver JL, Albers GW, Alberts MJ, Chaturvedi S, Feldmann E, et al. Definition and evaluation of transient ischemic attack: A scientific statement for healthcare professionals from the American Heart Association/ American Stroke Association Stroke Council; Council on Cardiovascular Surgery and Anesthesia; Council on Cardiovascular Radiology and Intervention; Council on Cardiovascular Nursing; and the Interdisciplinary Council on Peripheral VascularDisease. Stroke. 2009;**40**:2276-2293. DOI: 10.1161/STROKEAHA.108.192218

[4] Del Zoppo JD, Hallenbeck JM. Advances in the vascular pathophysiology of ischemic stroke. Thrombosis Research. 2000;**98**(3):73-81

[5] Helgason CM, Wolf PA. American heart association prevention conference IV: Prevention and rehabilitation of Stroke. Circulation. 1997;**96**:701-707. DOI: 10.1161/01.CIR.96.2.701

[6] Frizzell JP. Acute stroke: Pathophysiology, diagnosis, and treatment. AACN Clinical Issues: Advanced Practice in Acute and Critical Care. 2005;**16**(4):421-598

[7] Balci K, Utku U, Asil T, Unlu E. Simultaneous onset of hemorrhagic and ischemic strokes. The Neurologist. 2007;**13**(3):148-149

[8] Vermeer SE, Algra A, Franke CL, Koudstaal PJ, Rinkel GJE. Long-term prognosis after recovery from primary intracerebral hemorrhage. Neurology. 2002;**59**(2):205-209

[9] Mishra LD. Cerebral blood flow and anaesthesia. Indian Journal of Anaesthesia. 2002;**46**(2):87-95

[10] Kalogeris T, Baines CP, Krenz M, Korthuis RJ. Cell biology of ischemia/ reperfusion injury. International Review of Cell and Molecular Biology. 2012;**298**:229-317. DOI: 10.1016/ B978-0-12-394309-5.00006-7

[11] Sims NR, Anderson MF. Mitochondrial contributions to tissue damage in stroke. Neurochemistry International. 2002;**40**(6):511-526

[12] Deba P, Sharma S, Hassan KM. Pathophysiologic mechanisms of acute ischemic stroke: An overview with emphasis on therapeutic significance beyond thrombolysis. Pathophysiology. 2010;**17**:197-218. DOI: 10.1016/j. pathophys.2009.12.001

[13] Hachinski V, Iadecola C, Petersen C, Breteler MM, Nyenhuis DL, Black SE, et al. National institute of neurological disorders and stroke—Canadian stroke network vascular cognitive impairment harmonization standards. Stroke. 2006;**37**:2220-2241. DOI: 10.1161/01. STR.0000237236.88823.47

[14] World Heart Federation (WHF). Global Burden of Stroke [Internet]. 2017. Available from: http://www.world-heart-federation.org/cardiovascular-health/stroke/ [Accessed: May 25, 2018]

[15] Chong J, Sacco R, Ovbiagele B, Nguyen-Huynh MN. Stroke epidemiology: Advancing our

understanding of disease mechanism and therapy. Neurotherapeutics. 2011;**8**(3):319-329. DOI: 10.1007/s13311-011-0053-1

[16] O'Donnell MJ, Xavier D, Liu L, et al. Risk factors for ischaemic and intracerebral haemorrhagic stroke in 22 countries (The Interstroke Study): A case-control study. Lancet. 2010;**376**:112-123. DOI: 10.1016/S0140-6736(10)60834-3

[17] Petrea RE, Beiser AS, Seshadri S, Kelly-Hayes M, Kase CS, Wolf PA. Gender differences in stroke incidence and poststroke disability in the framingham heart study. Stroke. 2009;**40**:1032-1037. DOI: 10.1161/STROKEAHA.108.542894

[18] Niewada M, Kobayashi A, Sandercock PA, Kaminski B, Czlonkowska A. Influence of gender on baseline features and clinical outcomes among 17,370 patients with confirmed ischaemic stroke in the international stroke trial. Neuroepidemiology. 2004;**24**:123-128

[19] Pound P, Gompertz P, Ebrahim S. A patient-centred study of the consequences of stroke. Clinical Rehabilitation. 1998;**12**(4):338-347

[20] Shumway-Cook A, Woollacott MH. Motor Control: Theory and Practical Applications. 2nd ed. Philadelphia: Lippincott Williams & Wilkins; 2001

[21] Haas B. Motor Control. In: Everett T, Kell C, editors. Human Movement. Edinburgh: Churchill Livingstone; 2010. pp. 47-60

[22] Gerloff C, Corwell B, Chen R, Hallett M, Cohen LG. The role of the human motor cortex in the control of complex and simple finger movement sequences. Brain. 1998;**121**(Pt 9): 1695-1709

[23] Swenson RS. Chapter 11: The Cerebral Cortex. Review of Clinical and Functional Neuroscience [Internet]. 2006. Available from: https://www.dartmouth.edu/~rswenson/NeuroSci/ [Accessed: June 6, 2018]

[24] Lanciego JL. Basal ganglia circuits: what's now and next? Frontiers in Neuroanatomy. 2012;**6**:4. DOI: 10.3389/fnana.2012.00004

[25] Taub E, Berman AJ. Avoidance conditioning in the absence of relevant proprioceptive and exteroceptive feed back. Journal of Comparative and Physiological Psychology. 1963;**56**: 1012-1016. DOI: 10.1037/h0048315

[26] Ostendorf CG, Wolf SL. Effect of forced use of the upper extremity of a hemiplegic patient on changes in function: A single-case design. Physical Therapy. 1981;**61**(7):1022-1028. DOI: 10.1093/ptj/61.7.1022

[27] Taub E, Miller NE, Novack TA, Cook IEW, Fleming WC, Nepomuceno CS. Technique to improve chronic motor deficit after stroke. Archives of Physical Medicine and Rehabilitation. 1993;**74**(4):347-354

[28] Taub E, Uswatte G, King DK, Morris D, Crago JE, Chatterjee A. A placebo-controlled trial of constraint-induced movement therapy for upper extremity after stroke. Stroke. 2006;**37**(4):1045-1049

[29] Sunderland A, Tuke A. Neuroplasticity, learning and recovery after stroke: A critical evaluation of constraint-induced therapy. Neuropsychological Rehabilitation. 2005;**15**:81-98

[30] Wolf SL, Lecraw DE, Barton LA, Jann BB. Forced use of hemiplegic upper extremities to reverse the effect of learned nonuse among chronic stroke and head-injured patients. Experimental Neurology. 1989;**104**(2):125-132

[31] Wolf SL, Winstein CJ, Miller JP, Taub E, Uswatte G, Morris D. Effect of constraint-induced movement therapy on upper extremity function 3 to 9 months after stroke: The EXCITE randomized clinical trial. JAMA. 2006;**296**(17):2095-2104. DOI: 10.1001/jama.296.17.2095

[32] Okamoto H, Fukushima M, Teismann H, Lagemann L, Kitahara T, Inohara H, et al. Constraint-induced sound therapy for sudden sensorineural hearing loss—Behavioral and neurophysiological outcomes. Scientific Reports. 2014;**4**:3927. DOI: 10.1038/srep03927

[33] Matuti GD-S, Pires CVG, Rafael Garcia RE, Oliveira CB. Constraint induced movement therapy in patients with incomplete tetraplegia after spinal cord injury. Archives of Physical Medicine and Rehabilitation. 2015;**96**(10):85-e86. DOI: 10.1016/j.apmr.2015.08.287

[34] Buesch FE, Schlaepfer B, de Bruin ED, Wohlrab G, Ammann-Reiffer C, Meyer-Heim A. Constraint-induced movement therapy for children with obstetric brachial plexus palsy: Two single-case series. International Journal of Rehabilitation Research. 2010;**33**(2):187-192. DOI: 10.1097/MRR.0b013e3283310d6e

[35] Mark VW, Taub E, Uswatte G, Morris DM, Cutter GR, Adams TL, et al. Phase II randomized controlled trial of constraint-induced movement therapy in multiple sclerosis. Part 1: Effects on real-world function. Neurorehabilitation and Neural Repair. 2018;**32**(3):223-232. DOI: 10.1177/1545968318761050

[36] Burkhardt J, Sheridan J, Villavecchia P, Hollander L, Garbarini JG. Effectiveness of constraint-induced movement therapy for functional use in children with spastic hemiplegic cerebral palsy: A systematic review. American Journal of Occupational Therapy. 2017;**71**:7111520311p1. DOI: 10.5014/ajot.2017.71S1-PO6088

[37] Mark VW, Taub E, Uswatte G, Bashir K, MD CGR, Bryson CC, et al. Constraint-induced movement therapy for the lower extremities in multiple sclerosis: Case series with 4-year follow-up. Archives of Physical Medicine and Rehabilitation. 2013;**94**:753-760. DOI: 10.1016/j.apmr.2012.09.032

[38] Etoom M, Hawamdeh M, Hawamdeh Z, et al. Constraint-induced movement therapy as a rehabilitation intervention for upper extremity in stroke patients: Systematic review and metaanalysis. International Journal of Rehabilitation Research. 2016;**39**(3):197-210. DOI: 10.1097/MRR.0000000000000169

[39] Morris DM, Taub E, Mark VW. Constraint-induced movement therapy: Characterizing the intervention protocol. Europa Medicophysica. 2006;**42**:257-268

[40] Kim H, Yoo EY, Jung MY, Kim J, Park JH, Kang DH. The effects of mental practice combined with modified constraint-induced therapy on corticospinal excitability, movement quality, function, and activities of daily living in persons with stroke. Disability and Rehabilitation. 2017;**9**:1-9. DOI: 10.1080/09638288.2017.1337817

[41] Taub E. The behaviour analytic origins of constraint-induced movement therapy: An example of behavioural neurorehabilitation. The Behaviour Analysis. 2012;**35**:155-178

[42] Wolf SL. Revisiting constraint-induced movement therapy: Are we too smitten with the mitten? is all nonuse "learned"? and other quandaries. Physical Therapy. 2007;**87**(9):1212-1223. DOI: 10.2522/ptj.20060355

[43] Taub E, Uswatte G, Mark VW, Morris DM, Barman J, Bowman MH, et al. Method for enhancing real-world use of a more-affected arm in chronic stroke: The transfer package of CI therapy. Stroke. 2013;**44**(5):1383-1388. DOI: 10.1161/STROKEAHA.111.000559

[44] Brogårdh C, Vestling M, Sjölund BH. Shortened constrained induced movement therapy in subacute stroke-no effect of using a restraint: A randomized controlled study with independent observers. Journal of Rehabilitation Medicine. 2009;**41**:231-236

[45] Abdullahi A, Shehu S, Dantani BI. Feasibility of high repetitions of tasks practice during constraint induced movement therapy in an acute stroke patient. International Journal of Therapy and Rehabilitation. 2014;**21**(4):190-195. DOI: 10.12968/ijtr.2014.21.4.190

[46] Collin A, Grimee M, Libois PY. The actimetry as assessment method of patients' compliance and effectiveness of constraint induced movement therapy. Annals of Physical and Rehabilitation Medicine. 2015;**58**(1):e8-e9

[47] Abu Taria H, Almalty A-M, Sbeih Z, Al-Oraib S. Constraint induced movement therapy for stroke survivors in Jordon: A home-based model. International Journal of Therapy and Rehabilitation. 2010;**17**(12):638-646. DOI: 10.12968/ijtr.2010.17.12.638

[48] Abdulahi A. Number of repetitions as measure of dose of shaping practice in acute stroke: Preliminary results of a randomized controlled trial. Neurorehabilitation and Neural Repair. 2018;**32**(4-5):402-403. DOI: 1177/1545968318765498

[49] Abdullahi. Effects of number of repetitions and number of hours of shaping practice during constraint-induced movement therapy: A randomized controlled trial. Neurology Research International. 2018. DOI: 10.1155/2018/5496408

[50] Lum PS, Taub E, Schwandt D, Postman M, Hardin P, Uswatte G. Automated constraint-induced therapy extension (AutoCITE) for movement deficits after stroke. Journal of Rehabilitation Research and Development. 2004;**41**(3A):249-258

[51] Viana R, Teasell R. Barriers to the implementation of constraint-induced movement therapy into practice. Topics in Stroke Rehabilitation. 2012;**19**(2):104-114. DOI: 10.1310/tsr1902-104

[52] Kaplon RT, Prettyman MG, Kushi CL, Winstein CJ. Six hours in the laboratory: Quantification of practice time during constraint induced therapy. Clinical Rehabilitation. 2007;**21**(10):950-958. DOI: 10.1177/0269215507078333

[53] Stock R, Thrane G, Askim T. Norwegian constraint-induced therapy multisite trial: Adherence to treatment protocol applied early after stroke. Journal of Rehabilitation Medicine. 2015;**47**:816-823

[54] Nijland R, Kwakkel G, Bakers J, van Wegen E. Constraint-induced movement therapy for the upper paretic limb in acute or sub-acute stroke: A systematic review. International Journal of Stroke. 2011;**6**(5):425-433. DOI: 10.1212/WNL.0b013e3181ab2b27

[55] Dromerick AW, Lang CE, Birkenmeier RL, Wagner JM, Miller JP, Videen TO, et al. Very early constraint-induced movement during stroke rehabilitation (VECTORS): A single-center RCT. Neurology. 2009;**73**(3):195-201

[56] Birkenmeier RL, Prager EM, Lang CE. Translating animal doses of task-specific training to people

with chronic stroke in 1-hour therapy sessions: A proof-of-concept study. Neurorehabilitation and Neural Repair. 2010;**24**(7):620-635. DOI: 10.1177/1545968310361957

[57] Ballester BR, Maier M, San Segundo MR-M, Castañeda V, Duff A, Verschure PFMJ. Counteracting learned non-use in chronic stroke patients with reinforcement-induced movement therapy. Journal of NeuroEngineering and Rehabilitation. 2016;**13**:74. DOI: 10.1186/s12984-016-0178-x

[58] Abdullahi A, Shehu S, Abdurrahman Z, Bello B. Determination of optimal dose of tasks practice during constraint induced movement therapy in a stroke patient with severe upper limb pain. Indian Journal of Physiotherapy and Occupational Therapy—An International Journal. 2015;**9**(1):198. DOI: 10.5958/0973-5674.2015.00039.8

[59] El-Helow MR, Zamzam ML, Fathalla MM, et al. Efficacy of modified constraint-induced movement therapy in acute stroke. European Journal of Physical and Rehabilitation Medicine. 2015;**51**(4):371-379

[60] Yu C, Wang W, Zhang Y, et al. The effects of modified constraintinduced movement therapy in acute subcortical cerebralinfarction. Frontiers in Human Neuroscience. 2017;**11**:265. DOI: 10.3389/fnhum.2017.00265

[61] Ro T, Noser E, Boake C, et al. Functional reorganization and recovery after constraint-induced movement therapy in subacute stroke: Case reports. Neurocase. 2006;**12**:50-60. DOI: 10.1080/13554790500493415

[62] Wu CY, Lin KC, Chen HC, Chen IH, Hong WH. Effects of modified constraint-induced movement therapy on movement kinematics and daily function in patients with stroke: A kinematic study of motor control mechanisms. Neurorehabilitation and Neural Repair. 2007;**21**(5):460-466

[63] Page SJ, Sisto S, Johnston HV, Levine P. Modified constraintinduced therapy after subacute stroke. Neurorehabilitation and Neural Repair. 2002;**16**:290-295

[64] Abdullahi A. Neurophysiological effects of constraint-induced movement therapy and motor function: A systematic review. International Journal of Therapy and Rehabilitation. 2018;**25**(4):167-176. DOI: 10.12968/ijtr.2018.25.4.167

[65] Abdullahi A. Upper limb self-efficacy test (UPSET): A measure of confidence in the use of upper limb after stroke. Advances of Science for Medicine. 2016;**1**(2):10-18

[66] Lin J-H, Hsu M-J, Sheu C-F. Psychometric comparisons of 4 measures for assessing upper-extremity function in people with stroke. Physical Therapy in Sport. 2009;**89**(8):840-850

[67] Wolf SL, Catlin PA, Ellis M, Archer AL, Morgan B, Piacentino A. Assessing wolf motor function test as outcome measure for research in patients after stroke. Stroke. 2001;**32**(7):1635-1639

[68] Uswatte G, Taub E, Morris D, Vignolo M, McCulloch K. Reliability and validity of the upper-extremity motor activity log-14 for measuring real-world arm use. Stroke. 2005;**36**(11):2493-2496

[69] vanderLee JH, Beckerman H, Knol DL, DeVet HCW, Boute LM. Clinimetric properties of the motor activity log for the assessment of arm use in hemiparetic patients. Stroke. 2004;**35**(6):1410-1414

[70] Zittel S, Weiller C, Liepert J. Citalopram improves dexterity in chronic stroke patients. Neurorehabilitation and Neural Repair. 2008;**22**(3):311-314

[71] Dobkin BH, Firestine A, West M. Ankle dorsiflexion as an fMRI paradigm to assay motor control for walking during rehabilitation. NeuroImage. 2004;**23**:370-381

[72] Sawaki L, Butler AJ, Leng X, Wassenaar PA, Mohammad YM, Blanton S, et al. Differential patterns of cortical reorganization following constraint-induced movement therapy during early and lateperiod after stroke: A preliminary study. Neurorehabilitation. 2014;**35**(3): 415-426. DOI: 10.3233/NRE-141132

[73] Cunningham DA, Varnerin N, Machado A, Bonnetta C, Janini D, Roelle S, et al. Stimulation targeting higher motor areas in stroke rehabilitation: A proof-of-concept, randomized, double-blinded placebo-controlled study of effectiveness and underlying mechanisms. Restorative Neurology and Neuroscience. 2015;**33**(6):911-926. DOI: 10.3233/RNN-150574

[74] Braun SM, Beurskens AJ, Borm PJ, Schack T, Derick Wade DT. The effects of mental practice in stroke rehabilitation: A systematic review. Archives of Physical Medicine and Rehabilitation. 2006;**87**(6):842-852. DOI: 10.1016/j.apmr.2006.02.034

[75] Kaya T, Karatepe AG, Gunaydin R, et al. Inter-rater reliability of the modified ashworth scale and modified modified ashworth scale in assessing poststroke elbow flexor spasticity. International Journal of Rehabilitation Research. 2011;**34**:59-64

[76] Korpershoek CL, van der Bijl J, Hafsteinsdottir TB. Self-efficacy and its influence on recovery of patients with stroke: A systematic review. Journal of Advanced Nursing. 2011;**67**(9):1876-1894. DOI: 10.1111/j.1365-2648.2011.05659.x

[77] Jones F, Riazi A. Self-efficacy and self-management after stroke: A systematic review. Disability and Rehabilitation. 2011;**33**(10):797-810. DOI: 10.3109/09638288.2010.511415

[78] Baker SE, Painter EE, Morgan BC. Systematic clinical reasoning in physical therapy (SCRIPT): Tool for the purposeful practice of clinical reporting in orthopaedic manual therapy. Physical Therapy. 2017;**97**:61-70

Chapter 3

Postural Control in Individuals with Parkinson's Disease

Marialuisa Gandolfi, Nicola Valè, Mirko Filippetti, Eleonora Kirilova Dimitrova, Christian Geroin, Alessandro Picelli and Nicola Smania

Abstract

Parkinson's disease is the second most common neurodegenerative disorder in the elderly population. It is a complex, progressive, multisystem disease associated with motor and nonmotor impairments. Postural instability is a crucial component of functional mobility, often overlooked by both clinicians and patients with Parkinson's disease. It is a refractory drug complication for which rehabilitation is the most effective nonpharmacological aid. However, many interventions are based on empirical experience. Improving knowledge on the pathophysiology of postural control disorders is crucial to understand the multifaceted components affected and thus design specific rehabilitation protocols. This chapter intends to offer a comprehensive overview of the current knowledge on this topic starting from the pathophysiology of postural control disorders occurring in various ecological conditions to the most innovative multidisciplinary rehabilitation approaches.

Keywords: postural balance, accidental falls, neurological gait dysfunction, neurological rehabilitation, virtual reality, robotics

1. Introduction

Postural control is a key component for the safety performance of daily activities. Specifically, the control of posture is essential to stabilize the body's center of mass (COM) relative to the base of support and for the proper alignment of the body with the body's center of gravity (COG), the support surface, and the surrounding environment. Moreover, it facilitates performance of a manual task. Postural control disturbances and resulting falls are significant factors determining the quality of life (QOL), morbidity, and mortality [1].

Parkinson's disease (PD) is the second most common neurodegenerative disorder affecting 2–3% of the population over 65 years of age [2]. Neuronal loss in the substantia nigra causes striatal dopamine deficiency and intracellular inclusions containing aggregates of α-synuclein that are the neuropathological hallmarks of PD. Multiple other cell types throughout the central and peripheral and autonomic nervous systems are also involved, probably from the disease onset. The clinical diagnosis relies on the presence of bradykinesia and other cardinal motor features such as rigidity, postural instability, and tremor. However, PD is associated with motor and nonmotor symptoms that add to overall disability and increase the risk of postural control disturbances.

Postural control disturbances are one of the most common challenging signs in PD and one of the main concerns in rehabilitation. According to a fall retrospective study, falls are a significant problem for older people with PD as well as younger ones with advanced stages of the disease [3]. Up to 68.3% of people with PD fall each year, with around 50% reporting recurrent falls [4]. The most frequent consequences of falling are injuries [5] and fear of falling (FOF), both of which limit physical activity and lower QOL [6, 7]. Several factors have been associated with recurrent falls in PD, including a positive fall history, disease severity and duration, motor disturbances, medications, cognitive impairment, FOF, freezing of gait (FOG), impaired mobility, and reduced physical activity [8].

Rehabilitation has been considered as a crucial adjuvant to pharmacological and surgical treatments in PD to improve postural control, maximize the quality of life, and minimize secondary complications. However, many rehabilitation approaches are based on empirical experience and lack of knowledge of the underlying pathological mechanisms.

This chapter intends to offer a comprehensive overview of the current knowledge on this topic starting from the pathophysiology of postural control disorders occurring in various ecological conditions to the most innovative multidisciplinary rehabilitation approaches.

2. Pathophysiology of postural control

Postural control has two main functional goals: postural orientation and postural equilibrium. The former involves the active control of body alignment and tone to gravity, support surface, the visual environment, and internal references [9]. It is based on the interpretation of convergent sensory information from somatosensory, vestibular, and visual systems [10]. The latter refers to the coordination of sensorimotor strategies to stabilize the body's COM within the limits of stability imposed by the base of support during self-initiated and externally triggered tasks [10]. Body orientation and stabilization are distinct sensorimotor processes, and both are critical factors in preventing falls.

The postural control system consists of many subcomponents that may be grouped into six main domains: biomechanical constraints, movement strategies (i.e., reactive, anticipatory, and voluntary), sensory strategies (i.e., sensory integration and reweighting), orientation in space (i.e., perception, gravity, vision, and verticality), control of dynamics (i.e., gait and proactive), and cognitive processing (i.e., attention and executive functions) (**Figure 1**). A disorder in any of these resources may lead to postural instability and increase the risk of falling.

The assessment of postural control is crucial to determine specific deficits in the different subcomponents and to assess fall risk. In particular, instrumental assessment plays a threefold role: (1) understanding the pathophysiology of the postural control system, (2) defining clinical diagnosis, and (3) evaluating treatment efficacy. Among instruments, quantitative posturography is one of the most useful tools [11] because it can be performed during static and dynamic tasks as well as under different sensory conditions [11–13]. Other instruments for quantitative measurements of balance are stereophotogrammetric devices to measure the whole body movements through the detection of retroreflective markers, the pedobarography walkways to acquire spatial-temporal features of gait, and wearable inertial sensors (WIS) incorporating advanced electronic technologies to monitor functional activities (i.e., sensorized insoles to detect plantar pressures) [13].

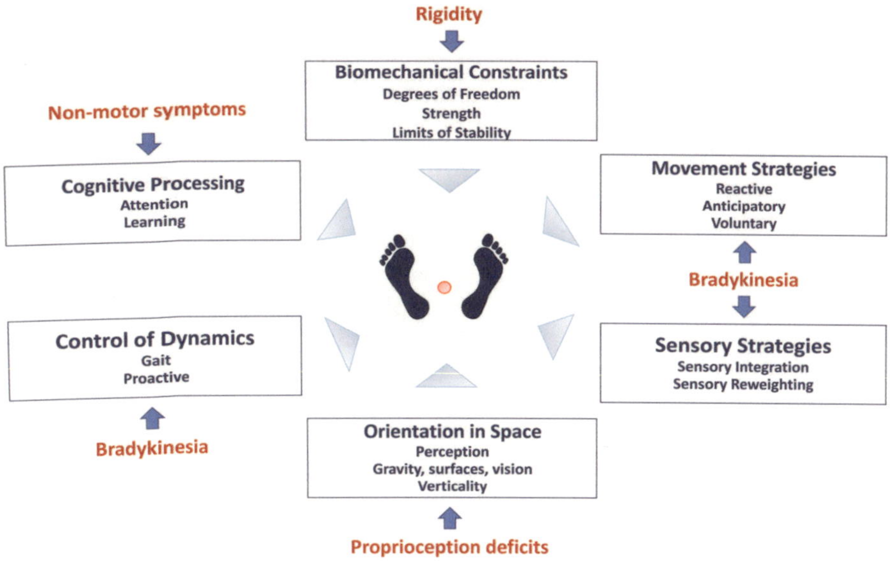

Figure 1.
Resources required for postural control.

3. Postural control during static tasks

Quiet stance is considered the result of automatic mechanisms working to some extent independently of cerebral cortical control. Postural sway in quiet stance appears to be increased in the elderly [14]. Patients with PD complain of abnormal postural sway even in the early stages of the disease [15–17]. They have increased postural sway, predominantly in the mediolateral direction. Center of pressure (COP) displacement is more significant in the lateral direction and is generally higher in velocity and frequency than in healthy subjects. Increased mediolateral COP displacement has been associated with an increased risk of falling [18, 19].

With eyes closed in the quiet stance, COP displacement is increased in the majority of healthy people, but it is markedly increased in patients with PD [15, 16]. The weaker performance of PD patients suggests that movement strategies and sensory integration deficits are both involved in these automatic tasks that also involve cognitive control and higher order cortical function [20]. For example, PD patients performing a cognitive and motor task in a quiet stance (dual-task condition) show increased sway velocity and area. Dyskinesia might contribute to the increased postural sway in patients with the more advanced stage of the disease, and this may contribute, at least in part, to the higher risk of falling that advanced PD patients experience during ON [21, 22].

Interesting results have been obtained with brain stimulation techniques. Pallidotomy and deep brain stimulation (DBS) of the globus pallidus internus may reduce postural sway, whereas conflicting results after subthalamic nucleus DBS have been reported [17, 23].

3.1 Biomechanical constraints

Several biomechanical constraints can affect balance: the base of support, the degree of joint freedom, limits of stability, and muscle strength [10]. The base of support is defined as the horizontal stride width in the double-support condition, with the feet in contact with the floor and the center of gravity (COG) within feet [24]. The limits of stability refer to the maximal excursion of the COM in different directions without changing the base of support (e.g., taking a step or falling). The central nervous system (CNS) has an internal representation of the limits of stability, which it uses to define the amplitude of movements to maintain balance. Basal ganglia dysfunction in patients with PD results in an abnormal representation of these limits of stability leading to postural control disorders [10]. In quiet stance, PD patients have an altered perception of these limits and display slower movement toward the limits, especially in the forward direction [25]. This slowness of COM movements has been related to the fear of falling (FOF) [7]. As to pharmacological treatments, levodopa therapy has been demonstrated to increase the perception of limits of stability and the velocity of COM displacement [25].

Muscle strength deficits along with muscle imbalance (i.e., muscle cocontraction) are important determinants of postural control disorders in PD. These impairments have rarely been investigated [26–30]. Although the specific causes of muscle weakness in PD are unknown and not explicitly related to tremor or rigidity, central and peripheral mechanisms might be put forward. Finally, whether muscle weakness is intrinsic to the disease or a secondary phenomenon is still under debate [28]. Inkster et al. [27] investigated the maximal concentric isokinetic knee and hip extensor torque in 10 men with mild PD using an isokinetic dynamometer. Data were compared with normative values collected in 10 sex- and age-matched controls. The PD patients were tested in both ON- and OFF-medication state on different days. The data showed that mean hip and knee extensor torques were lower in the PD patients, with more significant deficits at the hip. Greater hip strength was related to better sit-to-stand (STS) ability in the PD patients, whereas greater knee strength was related to better STS ability in the controls.

Durmus et al. [29] measured lower limb isokinetic muscle strength to investigate whether weakness in specific muscle may be associated with clinical severity and falls in 25 patients diagnosed with PD and 24 healthy volunteers.

A significant decrease in isokinetic muscle strength measured using an isokinetic dynamometer was observed in the PD patients, especially in the hip and knee flexors and extensors. Decreased muscle strength was independent of velocity but correlated with clinical severity and falls.

Allen et al. [26] investigated the relationship between leg extensor muscle power (i.e., the product of strength and speed of muscle contraction as a measure of the ability to use muscles quickly) and strength and the association with past falls and walking in 40 PD patients with mild-to-moderate PD. Patients with low muscle power were 6 times more likely to report multiple falls in the past 12 months than those with high muscle power. Although the association between falls and power was no longer significant after adjusting for the Unified Parkinson's Disease Rating Scale (UPDRS) motor score, muscle power was more strongly associated with past falls than muscle strength. This suggests that not only the force of contraction but also the velocity at which it can be generated determines the ability to perform physical activities and to recover from a loss of balance to prevent falls.

The importance of isokinetic muscle strength and power evaluation as a useful tool in the assessment of clinical severity and falls in PD has been emphasized [29–31]. Muscle power, muscle strength, and bradykinesia are potential targets for physical therapy interventions.

3.2 Movement strategies

Three postural strategies can be distinguished: ankle strategies, hip strategies, and stepping strategies. The ankle strategy refers to movements at the ankles in response to backward and forward tilt involving the distal muscles such as the tibialis anterior and the gastrocnemius muscles, respectively. This strategy is generally implemented to counteract small perturbations leaving feet in place (without the base of support enlargement).

The hip strategy consists of quick movements at the hip to maintain uprightness in more precarious conditions. Finally, the stepping strategy is used when perturbations occur or before reaching the limits of stability to return the COM to within the base of support. This strategy requires taking a step to enlarge the base of support. Together with these movement strategies, upper limb reactions may be employed to increase the limits of stability. In healthy subjects, the latency of the ankle and hip strategies is shorter (100 ms) than the stepping strategy (250 ms) [32]. In a quiet stance, the increase in mediolateral sway reflects decreasing postural control at the hip, whereas control in the anteroposterior direction is mainly related to activation of the ankle strategy [16]. Individuals with higher risk use the hip strategy more than those with a lower risk who use mainly ankle strategies.

Patients with PD have slower postural responses when in the OFF medication state [33]. Slowed postural adjustment induces a delay in returning of COM within the base of support, which exposes the patient to a higher risk of falling. Abnormal muscle activation such as cocontraction and short-duration bursting might further impair postural responses in PD [33, 34]. In the early stage of PD, balance is asymmetrically controlled in some patients with PD with the less affected leg producing more corrective joint torque than the other leg to maintain postural control [35]. Balance performance was evaluated in 20 PD patients and 11 healthy matched controls during 2 independent continuous multiline perturbations in the forward-backward direction. Applying closed-loop system identification techniques, relating the body sway angle to the joint torques of each leg separately, the investigators measured the relative contribution of each ankle and hip joint to the total amount of joint torque. The controls exhibited symmetric balance control. In contrast, the balance contribution of the less affected leg was higher than that of the leg of the more affected side in PD patients. The ratio between the legs helped to preserve a standard motor output at the ankle. These results suggest that PD patients compensate for postural control asymmetries by increasing the relative contribution of the less affected leg. This compensation appears to be successful at the ankle but is accompanied by increased stiffness at the hip [35]. Besides, other components such as intention, experience, and expectation can influence the movement strategy selection and the magnitude of postural responses [36].

Because of the impairment in the stepping strategy, patients with PD are unable to take steps wide enough to keep COM displacement within the base of support and so take additional steps. However, because such protective steps may not be significant enough to arrest movement of the COM, new stepping produces propulsion (if the COM is displaced forward) or retropulsion (if the COM is displaced backward). While healthy individuals take a compensatory step with no or only one anticipatory postural response, PD patients, especially those with freezing of gait (FOG), are often noted to make several anticipatory postural adjustments before stepping [37]. This delayed execution of the step is associated with "trembling of the knees" and increases the risk of falls [38]. Similar to voluntary steps, the size of automatically triggered protective stepping responses is improved by visual cues [39].

Postural abnormalities in PD are drug-refractory complications that affect postural reaction for balance maintenance [10]. The pathological underpinnings of camptocormia, antecollis, Pisa syndrome, and scoliosis have not yet been fully characterized, but either central or peripheral mechanisms might be the reasons for such deformities. Central mechanisms, such as trunk and lower limb muscle dystonia, may play a crucial role. Electromyography (EMG) studies in patients with PD and the Pisa syndrome [40–42] have shown greater activation of the paraspinal and nonparaspinal muscles bilaterally (cocontraction), ipsilateral or contralateral to trunk leaning or in camptocormia at the abdominal wall muscles than in healthy subjects. Peripheral mechanisms, such as myopathy and degenerative spinal and soft tissue changes, may all lead to muscle imbalance, weakness, and compensatory posture [43].

So far, the presumed effect of posture misalignments in postural control (i.e., Pisa syndrome) has been partially elucidated. Recent data indicate that the Pisa syndrome is associated with abnormal postural responses to maintain postural uprightness with significantly higher body sway velocity in the anteroposterior and mediolateral directions [44]. It means that a misalignment of posture may negatively influence postural and balance responses in PD patients and may be further comprised in patients unaware of their misalignment.

3.3 Sensory strategies

The ability of the CNS to use vestibular, somatosensory, and visual inputs to create a system of coordinates on which the body's postural control is based [45] is crucial to maintaining uprightness. In quite stance, healthy subjects rely on somatosensory (70%), vestibular (20%), and visual (10%) system inputs [46].

Sensory reweighting refers to the ability of the nervous system to integrate the different sources of information as well as changes in the surrounding environment. It means that sensory integration deficits may be related not only to dysfunction at the source but also to the ability to quickly change sensory weighting in different conditions (i.e., eyes open, eyes closed, and altered feet contact surface). Patients in the more advanced stage of PD have difficulty in maintaining uprightness on unstable surfaces with eyes closed [19], which is probably also related to a significant reduction in incoming proprioception information [47].

Finally, PD patients with posture misalignment might rely mostly on visual inputs to control their posture and postural reactions [44].

3.4 Orientation in space

Body alignment is defined as the relationship between body parts to one another and the ability to orient them to gravity, the base of support, and the surrounding environment. The nervous system in healthy humans is automatically able to modify body orientation in space according to the task and context in which a person is involved. In an experimental dark condition, healthy individuals can identify the gravitational vertical within 0.5° [10] according to multiple neural representations of verticality, or uprightness [48].

A tilted or inaccurate internal representation of verticality may affect postural alignment about gravity and lead to postural disorders. An altered sense of verticality in PD patients has been related to an impairment of the proprioceptive and somatosensory integration system [49], which affects the position of the body's COM over the base of support and makes patients more vulnerable to falls. Whether postural misalignment in PD (i.e., camptocormia, Pisa syndrome, antecollis, and scoliosis) depends on the inaccurate internal representation of verticality is still under investigation [50].

4. Postural control during dynamic tasks

The central nervous system uses compensatory postural adjustments (CPAs) and anticipatory postural adjustments (APAs) to maintain balance during dynamic and goal-oriented tasks [10] (**Figure 2**).

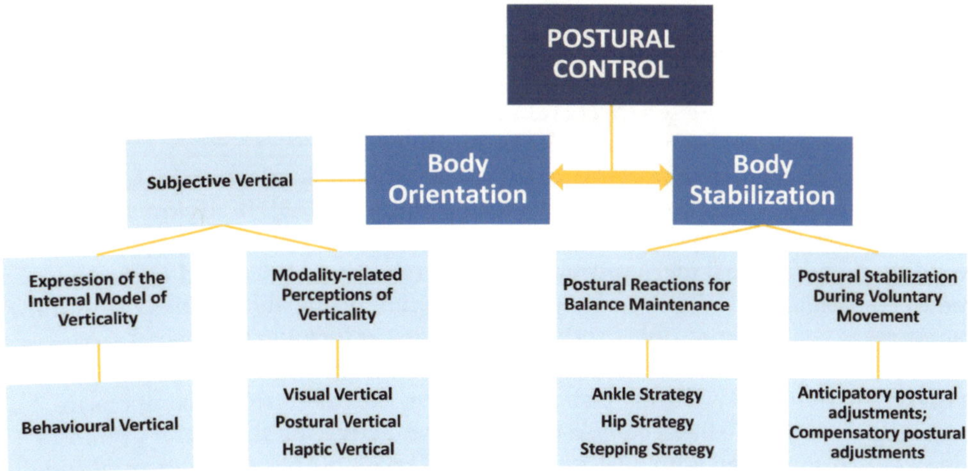

Figure 2.
Sensorimotor processes involved in postural control.

The former serves to restore the position of COM after a perturbation has occurred [32, 51]. CPAs rely mostly on the somatosensory and vestibular systems to determine the extent and type of perturbation and then to trigger the proper postural strategies. These postural responses are spinal and supraspinal polysynaptic responses and triggered by the difference between the actual and planned ankle joint trajectories [52].

The latter serves to minimize displacement of the COM before a perturbation [51–53]. Usually, APAs are associated with voluntary movements to reduce the effects of forthcoming disturbances by predicting the disturbance onset [53]. Another mode of APA control refers to the capability to detect potential environmental hazards and to implement the right postural adjustment before the risk event. In this context, vision and attention are critical factors in the early detection of potential balance threats, whereas complex sensorimotor integration processes are initiated to modify walking behavior to prevent falls promptly [54].

CPAs and APAs are thought to be involved in forming the so-called internal model, which is the internal representation of "motor and sensory signals related to a specific motor execution" [55]. An "internal model" exists for both the upper and the lower limbs [56]. In the lower limbs, the model adjusts for postural perturbation and novel dynamic environments during walking. Electrophysiological studies have emphasized that a combination of abnormal CPAs and APAs contributes to postural control disturbances in PD [57].

Different control mechanisms are involved during a static and dynamic task. However, postural control and active tasks are tightly intertwined. Significant insights into this topic have been gained from studies employing a battery of complementary research techniques, including electrophysiological techniques, and detailed postural control clinical evaluations (i.e., posturography) during dynamic tasks.

The sit-to-stand task, for instance, requires mainly APAs to displace the COM over the base of support before planning the sequence of movements to raise the body from a chair [58]. The inability of PD patients to perform this task may depend on altered APAs that do not allow bringing the COM adequately forward over the feet before the liftoff from a chair. In the early stage of the disease, patients show exaggerated movement preparation when performing the sit-to-stand tasks [59], whereas in the more advanced disease stages, reduced APAs have been measured [60].

Locomotion can be seen, in fact, as a four-step repeated sequence of balance challenges: gait initiation and generation of continuous movements to move forward and maintenance of postural equilibrium during progression; adaptability to any changes in the environment or other simultaneous tasks; gait termination [52]. Locomotion involves an intricate interplay between environmental conditions, goals, biomechanical constraints, sensory integration processes, and cognitive resources [61, 62]. All these aspects (alone or in combination) are impaired in PD patients.

Latash et al. reported that APA deficit might reflect disorders in the fundamental processes of preparation and initiation of a motor act [63]. Bradykinesia, one of the cardinal manifestations of PD, results from a failure of basal ganglia output to reinforce the cortical mechanisms involved in the preparation and execution of motor commands [64]. The resulting cortical deficit primarily involves the midline motor areas and is responsible for the difficulty in performing self-paced movements, for prolonged reaction times, and abnormal premovement electroencephalographic activity [64]. During task performance, the brain tries to compensate to some degree for the basal ganglia deficit by overactivating the lateral premotor areas. When compared with healthy subjects, PD patients have a lower amplitude of premotor potential during self-initiated movements, and underactivation of the supplementary motor area, anterior cingulate, left putamen, left insular cortex, right dorsolateral prefrontal cortex, and right parietal areas [65]. In contrast, no significant differences in early premotor potentials were found between PD patients and healthy subjects when externally triggered movements were performed. These findings confirm that the deficit in self-initiated movements in PD depends on the midline motor areas under activation and explain why movements can be speeded by sensory cues [66, 67].

Gait initiation refers to the capability to activate APAs that are essential to unload the swing leg and create the conditions for progression according to a highly stereotypical preparation muscle pattern activation. Moreover, the APA amplitude and duration are predictive of the subsequent peak step velocity [68]. Gait initiation disturbances in PD consist of the delayed release of APAs and hypokinetic anticipatory (reduced scaling) and bradykinetic APAs (abnormal timing) [68]. The most severe forms of gait initiation are the FOG and other phenomena such as the "knee trembling," which have been recognized as a sign of impaired APAs in PD patients with FOG [38]. FOG is a debilitating phenomenon during which the subject is suddenly unable to start walking or continue to move forward. It is usually thought to occur in the late stage of PD, but it also occurs in the early stages of idiopathic PD. FOG has been defined as a paroxysmal phenomenon, and little is known about its physiopathology. The influence of emotion, attention, external triggers, and dopaminergic drugs on gait initiation disturbances suggests the existence of multifactorial pathophysiology involving multiple nervous networks.

The generation of continuous movements to move forward and the processing of load-related input by the spinal cord central pattern generators are impaired in PD patients. It is associated with a reduction of leg extensor muscle activation and an enhanced leg flexor activity in the stance phase [52]. This pattern is associated with greater tibialis anterior muscle activity during the swing phase of gait that might reflect the stronger control of stance and gait in these patients by the visual system. Visual information can substitute to some extent reduced proprioception [69] improving walking [62].

Adaptability and variability in gait are related to the increased risk of falling and the decline in mobility [70]. Patients with PD showed more variability in step length and step time during gait than healthy subjects and freezers have a higher spatial gait variability between freezing episodes [71]. Variability in stride-time intervals is related to dynamic postural control, and it is associated with activation in the medial sensorimotor cortices, as measured using functional near-infrared spectroscopy (fNIRS) system [72]. The variability in stride-time intervals while walking forward was correlated with maximum activation in the precentral gyrus and supplementary motor area. However, activation in these areas and superior parietal lobule was higher when the subjects walked backward than forward suggesting that backward walking is a challenging task to the nervous system as it controls the stepping pattern [72]. Stride-to-stride variability is markedly increased among PD patients with FOG as compared to those without FOG, indicating that the inability to control cadence may play an essential role in this debilitating phenomenon. The effects of the dopamine-mediated pathways on stride-to-stride regulation and the role of attentional processes are thought to trigger FOG.

Literature on gait termination disorders in PD is scant. PD patients have difficulties in anticipating future target motion, which may play a role for the mechanisms involved in changing direction during gait and gait termination [73]. In contrast, their capacity of building up an internal representation of continuous target motion remains unimpaired. It may explain the clinical effects of medical devices that use visual motion to improve gait initiation (e.g., "PD glasses"). Further studies on the clinical effects of gait termination are needed.

Other relevant tasks concern difficulty turning during gait. Turning is a significant contributor to mobility disability, falls, and reduced quality of life in patients with PD [74]. It requires a complex integration between functionally different control mechanisms characterized by an upweighting of vestibular inputs and anticipatory postural adjustments [75]. Turning is accomplished by a top-down temporal sequence of body segment rotations that begins with an anticipatory redirection of gaze (saccade) toward the new heading direction. Increasing evidence suggests that eye movement is critical for turning control and that when the eyes are constrained, or participants have difficulty making eye movements, steering control is disrupted [76]. It has been demonstrated that APAs can be affected by the turn angle, the pivot foot, and speed and that they occur during the prior step. Healthy subjects usually lean backward and sideward on the previous step in anticipation of the turn, suggesting that the motor system uses central control mechanisms to predict the required anticipatory adjustments and organizes body configuration by the movement goal [75]. Animal studies have demonstrated that the basal ganglia network is involved in the posture-kinetic changes associated with turning and orientating behavior and that even PD patients with mild clinical impairment and no significant abnormalities in linear walking may exhibit turning disturbances [77]. PD patients show increased turn duration, a higher number of steps to turn, and difficulty in changing motor patterns from a straight line to turning [78, 79] even if their ability to scale movement speed and amplitude appears to be preserved. Moreover, altered oculomotor control is responsible for fewer, slower, and smaller preparatory saccades approaching a turn. Visuospatial dysfunction plays a central role in gait disturbance in PD, especially when navigating through complex environments [80].

Specific movement deficits in PD can be classified into perpendicular deficits (taking more steps and shorter steps and an altered turn strategy) and axial deficits (segment rigidity, altered segment coordination and timing, reduced segment rotation, and the effects of altered posture). Furthermore, FOF influences turning metrics in PD patients rather than a positive fall history [81]. Therefore, the specific focus should be made to the assessment and rehabilitation of the axial deficits alongside those of the straight body segments in the design of multimodal treatment strategies to improve turning performance.

The relationship between cognitive function and balance "per se" has rarely been investigated. In contrast, a growing body of evidence indicated the role played by cognition in the control of gait. Gait is considered an activity that requires executive function, visuospatial abilities, memory resources, and attention as well as the judgment of external and internal cues. Some morphological and functional neuroimaging studies have offered evidence supporting the relationship between gait and cognitive resource functional neuroimaging studies.

5. Rehabilitation approaches

Patients with PD show impairments in many aspects of postural control including rigidity affecting biomechanical constraints, bradykinesia of postural adjustments, impaired sensory integration processes, and bradykinetic gait with freezing. Postural control disorders are disabling and drug-refractory complications in PD. In this context, rehabilitation is crucial to maximize functional ability and minimize secondary complications within the context of education and support. Rehabilitation can ameliorate postural control through practice and enables patients to benefit from exercises that challenge their gait and postural control. Initially, practical experience has driven the rehabilitation of postural control disorders. However, improvements in understanding the mechanisms underlying postural control disorders in PD have ultimately lead us to improve the management strategies.

Since the pathophysiology of postural control disorders is multifaceted, the different rehabilitative approaches proposed in literature should be combined in a comprehensive rehabilitation program addressing all the affected domains. Moreover, according to the disease stage, specific rehabilitation approaches should be proposed.

Patients and their family members should be advised on the importance of maintaining adequate motor activity to preserve motor function and prevent the decline in mobility starting soon after the diagnosis. At relatively early stages of the disease, the importance of home exercise routines such as Nordic walking, treadmill training, and balance training consisting of a combination of strengthening and balance exercises may lead to an improvement in self-perceived performance in daily activities and reduce the gradual decline in mobility [83–88]. At this stage, dance therapy and martial arts might improve significantly postural control with a decrease in falls [83] and offer the advantage of social engagement, from an ICF perspective. Exercises aimed at improving sensorimotor integration are crucial, and in the early stage of the disease, they can be carried out using virtual reality scenarios and exergaming. Virtual reality has emerged as a therapeutic tool facilitating motor learning for balance and gait rehabilitation [84] especially in the early stages of the disease as home rehabilitation interventions [85].

With the progression of the disease, home exercise routines need to be progressively supported by specific rehabilitation interventions delivered by health professionals. In the comprehensive management of patients with PD, the presence of limiting factors such as motor fluctuations (on/off phase), dyskinesia, fatigue, and the cognitive status should be taken into account. Previous reviews emphasized the role of exercises that challenge various PD-specific component of postural control including the stability limits, APAs, CPAs, and dynamic stability [82]. In the advanced stage of the disease, the rehabilitation of postural disorders might be enriched using technological devices. Robotic rehabilitation is a rapidly growing field of application. The primary advantage of using robot technologies is the possibility to deliver high-dosage and high-intensity training. A recent systematic review [83] analyzed safety, feasibility, and effectiveness of exergaming for PD and demonstrated that people with PD were able to play exergames, enjoyed playing, and showed some improvements in motor symptoms (balance). Furthermore, MI and AOT demonstrated potential benefit in PD patients because of improvement in motor skills by enhancing proprioceptive signals normally generated during movements and activation of the mirror neuron system, respectively [83].

Growing evidence has suggested that rehabilitation could induce long-lasting and clinically meaningful benefits, particularly for postural control and gait. These training effects may be associated with exercise-induced neuroplasticity phenomena by increasing synaptic strength and influencing neurotransmission [82].

To date, there is still no consensus about the optimal rehabilitation approach ought to an extensive heterogeneity of interventions (i.e., stretching, muscle strengthening, balance, postural exercises, occupational therapy, cueing, and treadmill training) [83]. Indeed, these interventions bring additional benefits when combined with "conventional rehabilitation" in the context of specific theory-driven protocols. The number of practice variables (i.e., duration, intensity, specificity, and complexity) needs to be tailored to the individual patients' characteristics. Besides, the interplay between higher-order neural function and postural control has many clinical implications, ranging from integrated assessment tools to possible innovative lines of interventions, including cognitive therapy for fall prevention on the one hand and walking program for reducing cognitive decline risk on the other.

6. Conclusion

The new knowledge on the effects of environment and task on postural control in individuals with Parkinson's disease is fascinating and emphasized the complicated interplay between cognitive and sensorimotor processes. Improvements in understanding these mechanisms have ultimately improved the management strategies in rehabilitation. To date, specific rehabilitation approaches can be selected according to the stage of the disease and the specific postural control impairment.

Appendices and nomenclature

APAs	anticipatory postural adjustments
CNS	central nervous system
COG	center of gravity
COM	center of mass
COP	center of pressure
CPAs	compensatory postural adjustments
DBS	deep brain stimulation
EMG	electromyography
fNIRS	functional near-infrared spectroscopy
FOF	fear of falling
FOG	freezing of gait
PD	Parkinson's disease
QOL	quality of life
STS	sit-to-stand

Author details

Marialuisa Gandolfi[1*], Nicola Valè[1], Mirko Filippetti[2], Eleonora Kirilova Dimitrova[1], Christian Geroin[1], Alessandro Picelli[1] and Nicola Smania[1]

1 Department of Neuroscience, Biomedicine and Movement Science, Neuromotor and Cognitive Rehabilitation Research Centre (CRRNC), University of Verona, Italy

2 School of Specialization in Physical Medicine and Rehabilitation, University of Verona, Italy

*Address all correspondence to: marialuisa.gandolfi@univr.it

References

[1] Schoneburg B, Mancini M, Horak F, Nutt JG. Framework for understanding balance dysfunction in Parkinson's disease. Movement Disorders. 2013;**28**:1474-1482

[2] Poewe W, Seppi K, Taner CM, Halliday GM, Brundin P, Volkmann J, et al. Parkinson disease. Nature Reviews Disease Primers. 2017;**23**:1-21

[3] Stolze H, Klebe S, Zechlin C, Baecker C, Friege L, Deuschl G. Falls in frequent neurological diseases: Prevalence, risk factors and aetiology. Journal of Neurology. 2004;**251**:79-84

[4] Wood BH, Bilclough JA, Bowron A, Walker RW. Incidence and prediction of falls in Parkinson's disease: A prospective multidisciplinary study. Journal of Neurology, Neurosurgery, and Psychiatry. 2002;**72**:721-725

[5] Temlett JA, Thompson PD. Reasons for admission to hospital for Parkinson's disease. Internal Medicine. 2006;**36**:524-526

[6] Adkin AL, Frank JS, Jog MS. Fear of falling and postural control in Parkinson's disease. Movement Disorders. 2003;**18**:496-502

[7] Franchignoni F, Martignoni E, Ferriero G, Pasetti C. Balance and fear of falling in Parkinson's disease. Parkinsonism & Related Disorders. 2005;**11**:427-433

[8] Allen NE, Schwarzel AK, Canning CG. Recurrent falls in Parkinson's disease: A systematic review. Parkinson's Disease. 2013;**906274**:1-16

[9] Amblard B, Crémieux J, Marchand AR, Carblanc A. Lateral orientation and stabilization of human stance: Static versus dynamic visual cues. Experimental Brain Research. 2015;**61**:21-37

[10] Horak FB. Postural orientation and equilibrium: What do we need to know about neural control of balance to prevent falls? Age and Ageing. 2006;(Suppl2):ii7-ii11

[11] Visser JE, Carpenter MG, van der Kooij H, Bloem BR. The clinical utility of posturography. Clinical Neurophysiology. 2008;**119**:2424-2436

[12] Perry J, Burnfield JM. Gait Analysis: Normal and Pathological Function. 2nd ed. New Jersey: SLACK Incorpored; 2010. 576 p

[13] Sandrini G, Homberg V, Saltuari L, Smania N, Pedrocchi A. Advanced Technologies for the Rehabilitation of Gait and Balance Disorders. Springer-Verlag; 2018. 536 p

[14] Ickenstein GW, Ambach H, Klöditz A, Koch H, Isenmann S, et al. Static posturography in aging and Parkinson's disease. Frontiers in Aging Neuroscience. 2012;**4**:20

[15] Mancini M, Horak FB, Zampieri C, Carlson-Kuhta P, Nutt JG, Chiari L. Trunk accelerometry reveals postural instability in untreated Parkinson's disease. Parkinsonism & Related Disorders. 2011;**17**(7):557-562

[16] Stylianou AP, McVey MA, Lyons KE, Pahwa R, Luchies CW. Postural sway in patients with mild to moderate Parkinson's disease. International Journal of Neuroscience. 2011;**121**:614-621

[17] Nantel J, McDonald JC, Bronte-Stewart H. Effect of medication and STN-DBS on postural control in subjects with Parkinson's disease. Parkinsonism & Related Disorders. 2012;**18**:285-289

[18] Matinolli M, Korpelainen JT, Korpelainen R, Sotaniemi KA, Virranniemi M, et al. Postural sway and falls in Parkinson's disease:

A regression approach. Movement Disorders. 2007;**22**:1927-1935

[19] Frenklach A, Louie S, Koop MM, Bronte-Stewart H. Excessive postural sway and the risk of falls at different stages of Parkinson's disease. Movement Disorders. 2009;**24**:377-385

[20] Marchese R, Bove M, Abbruzzese G. Effect of cognitive and motor tasks on postural stability in Parkinson's disease: A posturographic study. Movement Disorders. 2003;**18**:652-658

[21] Chung KA, Lobb BM, Nutt JG, McNames J, Horak F. Objective measurement of dyskinesia in Parkinson's disease using a force plate. Movement Disorders. 2010;**25**:602-608

[22] Ashburn A, Stack E, Pickering RM, Ward CD. A community-dwelling sample of people with Parkinson's disease: Characteristics of fallers and non-fallers. Age and Ageing. 2001;**30**:47-52

[23] Bronte-Stewart HM, Minn AY, Rodrigues K, Buckley EL, Nashner LM. Postural instability in idiopathic Parkinson's disease: The role of medication and unilateral pallidotomy. Brain. 2002;**125**:2100-2114

[24] Krebs DE, Goldvasser D, Lockert JD, Portney LG, Gill-Body KM. Is base of support greater in unsteady gait? Physical Therapy. 2002;**82**:138-147

[25] Mancini M, Rocchi L, Horak FB, Chiari L. Effects of Parkinson's disease and levodopa on functional limits of stability. Clinical Biomechanics (Bristol, Avon). 2008;**23**:450-458

[26] Allen NE, Canning CG, Sherrington C, Lord SR, Latt MD, et al. The effects of an exercise program on fall risk factors in people with Parkinson's disease: A randomized controlled trial. Movement Disorders. 2010;**25**:1217-1225

[27] Inkster LM, Eng JJ, MacIntyre DL, Stoessl AJ. Leg muscle strength is reduced in Parkinson's disease and relates to the ability to rise from a chair. Movement Disorders. 2003;**18**:157-162

[28] Cano-de-la-Cuerda R, Pérez-de-Heredia M, Miangolarra-Page JC, Muñoz-Hellín E, Fernández-de-Las-Peñas C. Is there muscular weakness in Parkinson's disease? American Journal of Physical Medicine & Rehabilitation. 2010;**89**:70-76

[29] Durmus B, Baysal O, Altinayar S, Altay Z, Ersoy Y, et al. Lower extremity isokinetic muscle strength in patients with Parkinson's disease. Journal of Clinical Neuroscience. 2010;**17**:893-896

[30] Paul SS, Canning CG, Sherrington C, Fung VS. Reduced muscle strength is the major determinant of reduced leg muscle power in Parkinson's disease. Parkinsonism & Related Disorders. 2012;**18**:974-977

[31] Tambosco L, Percebois-Macadré L, Rapin A, Nicomette-Bardel J, Boyer FC. Effort training in Parkinson's disease: A systematic review. Annals of Physical and Rehabilitation Medicine. 2014;**57**:79-104

[32] Horak FB, Nashner LM. Central programming of postural movements: Adaptation to altered support-surface configurations. Journal of Neurophysiology. 1986;**55**:1369-1381

[33] Horak FB, Frank J, Nutt J. Effects of dopamine on postural control in parkinsonian subjects: Scaling, set, and tone. Journal of Neurophysiology. 1996;**75**:2380-2396

[34] Hallett M, Khoshbin S. A physiological mechanism of bradykinesia. Brain. 1980;**103**:301-314

[35] Boonstra TA, Schouten AC, van Vugt JP, Bloem BR, van der Kooij H. Parkinson's disease patients compensate

for balance control asymmetry. Journal of Neurophysiology. 2014;**112**:3227-3239

[36] Burleigh AL, Horak FB, Malouin F. Modification of postural responses and step initiation: Evidence for goal-directed postural interactions. Journal of Neurophysiology. 1994;**72**:2892-2902

[37] King LA, St George RJ, Carlson-Kuhta P, Nutt JG, Horak FB. Preparation for compensatory forward stepping in Parkinson's disease. Archives of Physical Medicine and Rehabilitation. 2010;**91**:1332-1338

[38] Jacobs JV, Nutt JG, Carlson-Kuhta P, Stephens M, Horak FB. Knee trembling during freezing of gait represents multiple anticipatory postural adjustments. Experimental Neurology. 2009;**215**:334-341

[39] Jacobs JV, Horak FB. External postural perturbations induce multiple anticipatory postural adjustments when subjects cannot pre-select their stepping foot. Experimental Brain Research. 2007;**179**:29-42

[40] Tinazzi M, Juergenson I, Squintani G, Vattemi G, Montemezzi S, et al. Pisa syndrome in Parkinson's disease: An electrophysiological and imaging study. Journal of Neurology. 2013;**260**:2138-2148

[41] Di Matteo A, Fasano A, Squintani G, Ricciardi L, Bovi T, et al. Lateral trunk flexion in Parkinson's disease: EMG features disclose two different underlying pathophysiological mechanisms. Journal of Neurology. 2011;**258**:740-745

[42] Tassorelli C, Furnari A, Buscone S, Alfonsi E, Pacchetti C, et al. Pisa syndrome in Parkinson's disease: Clinical, electromyographic, and radiological characterization. Movement Disorders. 2012;**27**:227-235

[43] Ponfick M, Gdynia HJ, Ludolph AC, Kassubek J. Camptocormia in Parkinson's disease: A review of the literature. Neurodegenerative Diseases. 2011;**8**:283-288

[44] Geroin C, Smania N, Schena F, Dimitrova E, Verzini E, Bombieri F, et al. Does the Pisa syndrome affect postural control, balance, and gait in patients with Parkinson's disease? An observational cross-sectional study. Parkinsonism & Related Disorders. 2015;**21**(7):736-741

[45] Smania N, Picelli A, Gandolfi M, Fiaschi A, Tinazzi M. Rehabilitation of sensorimotor integration deficits in balance impairment of patients with stroke hemiparesis: A before/after pilot study. Neurological Sciences. 2008;**29**:313-319

[46] Peterka RJ, Benolken MS. Role of somatosensory and vestibular cues in attenuating visually induced human postural sway. Experimental Brain Research. 1995;**105**:101-110

[47] Konczak J, Corcos DM, Horak F, Poizner H, Shapiro M, et al. Proprioception and motor control in Parkinson's disease. Journal of Motor Behavior. 2009;**41**:543-552

[48] Karnath HO, Ferber S, Dichgans J. The neural representation of postural control in humans. PNAS. 2000;**97**:13931-13936

[49] Smania N, Corato E, Tinazzi M, Stanzani C, Fiaschi A, et al. Effect of balance training on postural instability in patients with idiopathic Parkinson's disease. Neurorehabilitation and Neural Repair. 2010;**24**:826-834

[50] Doherty KM, van de Warrenburg BP, Peralta MC, Silveira-Moriyama L, Azulay JP, et al. Postural deformities in Parkinson's disease. Lancet Neurology. 2011;**10**:538-549

[51] Alexandrov AV, Frolov AA, Horak FB, Carlson-Kuhta P, Park S. Feedback equilibrium control during human standing. Biological Cybernetics. 2005;**93**:309-322

[52] Dietz V. Spinal cord pattern generators for locomotion. Clinical Neurophysiology. 2003;**114**:1379-1389

[53] Kim SD, Allen NE, Canning CG, Fung VS. Postural instability in patients with Parkinson's disease. Epidemiology, pathophysiology and management. CNS Drugs. 2013;**27**:97-112

[54] Woollacott M, Shumway-Cook A. Attention and the control of posture and gait: A review of an emerging area of research. Gait & Posture. 2002;**16**:1-14

[55] Frey SH, Fogassi L, Grafton S, Picard N, Rothwell JC, et al. Neurological principles and rehabilitation of action disorders: Computation, anatomy, and physiology (CAP) model. Neurorehabilitation and Neural Repair. 2011;**25**:6S-20S

[56] Lam T, Anderschitz M, Dietz V. Contribution of feedback and feedforward strategies to locomotor adaptations. Journal of Neurophysiology. 2006;**95**:766-773

[57] St George RJ, Carlson-Kuhta P, Burchiel KJ, et al. The effects of subthalamic and pallidal deep brain stimulation on postural responses in patients with Parkinson disease. Journal of Neurosurgery. 2012;**116**:1347-1356

[58] Goulart FR, Valls-Solé J. Patterned electromyographic activity in the sit-to-stand movement. Clinical Neurophysiology. 1999;**110**:1634-1640

[59] Inkster LM, Eng JJ. Postural control during a sit-to-stand task in individuals with mild Parkinson's disease. Experimental Brain Research. 2004;**154**:33-38

[60] Bleuse S, Cassim F, Blatt JL, Labyt E, Bourriez JL, al e. Anticipatory postural adjustments associated with arm movement in Parkinson's disease: A biomechanical analysis. Journal of Neurology, Neurosurgery, and Psychiatry. 2008;**79**:881-887

[61] Amboni M, Barone P, Hausdorff JM. Cognitive contributions to gait and falls: Evidence and implications. Movement Disorders. 2013;**28**:1520-1533

[62] Earhart GM. Dynamic control of posture across locomotor tasks. Movement Disorders. 2013;**28**:1501-1508

[63] Latash ML, Aruin AS, Neyman I, Nicholas JJ. Anticipatory postural adjustments during self inflicted and predictable perturbations in Parkinson's disease. Journal of Neurology, Neurosurgery, and Psychiatry. 1995;**58**:326-334

[64] Berardelli A, Rothwell JC, Thompson PD, Hallett M. Pathophysiology of bradykinesia in Parkinson's disease. Brain. 2001;**124**:2131-2146

[65] Jahanshahi M, Jenkins IH, Brown RG, Marsden CD, Passingham RE, et al. Self-initiated versus externally triggered movements. I. An investigation using measurement of regional cerebral blood flow with PET and movement-related potentials in normal and Parkinson's disease subjects. Brain. 1995;**118**:913-933

[66] Cassimatis C, Liu KP, Fahey P, Bissett M. The effectiveness of external sensory cues in improving functional performance in individuals with Parkinson's disease: A systematic review with meta-analysis. International Journal of Rehabilitation Research. 2016;**39**(3):211-218

[67] Ginis P, Nackaerts E, Nieuwboer A, Heremans E. Cueing for people with Parkinson's disease with freezing of gait: A narrative review of the

state-of-the-art and novel perspectives. Annals of Physical and Rehabilitation Medicine. 2017

[68] Delval A, Tard C, Defebvre L. Why we should study gait initiation in Parkinson's disease. Neurophysiologie Clinique. 2014;**44**(1):69-76

[69] Pearson KG. Proprioceptive regulation of locomotion. Current Opinion in Neurobiology. 1995;5:786-791

[70] Brach JS, Perera S, Studenski S, Katz M, Hall C, Verghese J. Meaningful change in measures of gait variability in older adults. Gait & Posture. 2010;**31**:175-179

[71] Amarell M, Snijders AH, Florin E, El Q, Schönau E, Fink GR, et al. Gait and upper limb variability in Parkinson's disease patients with and without freezing of gait. Journal of Neurology. 2014;**261**(2):330-342

[72] Kurz MJ, Wilson TW, Arpin DJ. Stride-time variability and sensorimotor cortical activation during walking. Neuroimage. 2012;**59**(2):1602-1607

[73] Helmchen C, Pohlmann J, Trillenberg P, Lencer R, Graf J, Sprenger A. Role of anticipation and prediction in smooth pursuit eye movement control in Parkinson's disease. Movement Disorders. 2012;**27**(8):1012-1018

[74] Mancini M, El-Gohary M, Pearson S, McNames J, Schlueter H, Nutt JG, et al. Continuous monitoring of turning in Parkinson's disease: Rehabilitation potential. NeuroRehabilitation. 2015;**37**(1):3-10

[75] Xu D, Carlton LG, Rosengren KS. Anticipatory postural adjustments for altering direction during walking. Journal of Motor Behavior. 2004;**36**:316-326

[76] Pradeep Ambati VN, Murray NG, Saucedo F, Powell DW, et al. Constraining eye movement when redirecting walking trajectories alters turning control in healthy young adults. Experimental Brain Research. 2013;**226**:549-556

[77] Crenna P, Carpinella I, Rabuffetti M, Calabrese E, Mazzoleni P, et al. The association between impaired turning and normal straight walking in Parkinson's disease. Gait & Posture. 2007;**26**:172-178

[78] Huxham F, Baker R, Morris ME, Iansek R. Footstep adjustments used to turn during walking in Parkinson's disease. Movement Disorders. 2008;**23**:817-823

[79] Stack E, Ashburn A. Dysfunctional turning in Parkinson's disease. Disability and Rehabilitation. 2008;**30**:1222-1229

[80] Galna B, Lord S, Daud D, Archibald N, Burn D, et al. Visual sampling during walking in people with Parkinson's disease and the influence of environment and dual-task. Brain Research. 2012;**1473**:35-43

[81] Haertner L, Elshehabi M, Zaunbrecher L, Pham MH, Maetzler C, van Uem JMT, et al. Effect of fear of falling on turning performance in Parkinson's disease in the lab and at home. Frontiers in Aging Neuroscience. 2018;**10**:78

[82] Mak MK, Wong-Yu IS, Shen X, Chung CL. Long-term effects of exercise and physical therapy in people with Parkinson disease. Nature Reviews. Neurology. 2017;**13**(11):689-703

[83] Abbruzzese G, Marchese R, Avanzino L, Pelosin E. Rehabilitation for Parkinson's disease: Current outlook and future challenges. Parkinsonism & Related Disorders. 2016;**22**(Suppl 1): S60-S64

[84] Cano Porras D, Siemonsma P, Inzelberg R, Zeilig G, Plotnik M. Advantages of virtual reality in the rehabilitation of balance and gait: Systematic review. Neurology. 2018;**90**(22):1017-1025

[85] Gandolfi M, Geroin C, Dimitrova E, Boldrini P, Waldner A, Bonadiman S, et al. Virtual reality telerehabilitation for postural instability in Parkinson's disease: A multicenter, single-blind, randomized, controlled trial. BioMed Research International. 2017;**7962826**:1-11

[86] Morrone M, Miccinilli S, Bravi M, Paolucci T, Melgari JM, Salomone G, et al. Perceptive rehabilitation and trunk posture alignment in patients with Parkinson disease: A single blind randomized controlled trial. European Journal of Physical and Rehabilitation Medicine. 2016;**52**(6):799-809

[87] Picelli A, Varalta V, Melotti C, Zatezalo V, Fonte C, Amato S, et al. Effects of treadmill training on cognitive and motor features of patients with mild to moderate Parkinson's disease: A pilot, single-blind, randomized controlled trial. Functional Neurology. 2016;**31**(1):25-31

[88] Picelli A, Melotti C, Origano F, Neri R, Verzè E, Gandolfi M, et al. Robot-assisted gait training is not superior to balance training for improving postural instability in patients with mild to moderate Parkinson's disease: A single-blind randomized controlled trial. Clinical Rehabilitation. 2015;**29**(4):339-347

Chapter 4

Physical Rehabilitation in the Management of Symptomatic Adult Scoliosis

Shu-Yan Ng, Tsz-Ki Ho and Yin-Ling Ng

Abstract

Scoliosis is prevalent in elderlies over the age of 60. Of the different curve types, the thoracolumbar curve is the most common curve type operated upon, as it is associated with marked trunk shift and disability. Current physiotherapy treatments consist of electrotherapy, aquatic exercises, core-strengthening exercises, and dry needling. Outcome of these treatments has not been satisfactory. Long-term successful rate of conservative treatment of symptomatic adult scoliosis is low, as the treatment addresses symptoms but not the biomechanics involved in adult scoliosis. Recent studies have shown that physiotherapeutic scoliosis-specific exercises (PSSE) and bracing stabilized the curves in 80% of the subjects. Thus PSSE and bracing should be added to the standard physiotherapy care in the management of symptomatic adult scoliosis. For asymptomatic patients with thoracolumbar curve that has an increased risk of progression, PSSE should be considered as preventative exercises. Patients who do not respond to conservative treatments and have significant spinal stenosis should be referred for surgery.

Keywords: degenerative lumbar scoliosis, adult scoliosis, scoliosis-specific exercises, physical rehabilitation

1. Introduction

Adult scoliosis refers to spinal curvature in excess of 10° after skeletal maturity. Common causes include adult idiopathic scoliosis (ADIS) and degenerative lumbar scoliosis (DLS). ADIS has its onset in childhood or adolescent. Degenerative lumbar scoliosis (DLS) is an adult-onset scoliosis brought about by degeneration of facet joints.

The prevalence of adult scoliosis varies with age and studies, ranging from 8.3 to 68% [1–5]. Xu et al. evaluated 2395 subjects over the age of 40 and reported that 13.3% had degenerative lumbar scoliosis (DLS) [5]. The prevalence increases with age. For subjects over 80 years of age, the prevalence is 27.1% [5]. Kobayashi et al. evaluated 60 elder normal subjects over 12 years and reported the prevalence of adult scoliosis to be 36.3% [1]. Schwab et al. reported the highest prevalence of 68% in 75 patients over the age of 60 [4].

The curve prevalence is inversely proportional to the curve magnitude. Majority of the curve is less than 10°. The prevalence of 10°, 10–20°, and >20° curves was reported to be 64, 44, and 24%, respectively [6].

IntechOpen

Of the different curve patterns, the thoracolumbar scoliosis is associated with a higher prevalence of low back pain and functional impairment [7]. Also, these curves tend to progress. The rate of progression for lumbar or thoracolumbar single curve was 0.82/year (0.34–1.65°) for adult idiopathic scoliosis patients [8]. The rate of progression is higher for curve in excess of 30° [9–11]. This was supported by a recent study on the radiographic parameter risk factors of rapid progression in adolescents with Lenke V and VI idiopathic scoliosis [12]. The study showed that apical vertebral rotation ≥ III (according to the Nash-Moe classification), deviation of the apical vertebra ≥40 mm from the central sacral line in the lumbar curve, and a L5 tilt angle ≥10° (**Figure 1**) are associated with an increased risk of curve progression in adolescents [12].

Likewise, DLS tends to progress but irrespective of the Cobb angle (**Figure 2**) [8]. For patients with DLS, the rate of progression was 1.64°/year (0.77–3.82°) [8]. A study which followed up 200 subjects over 50 years of age for 5 years showed that 73% of the

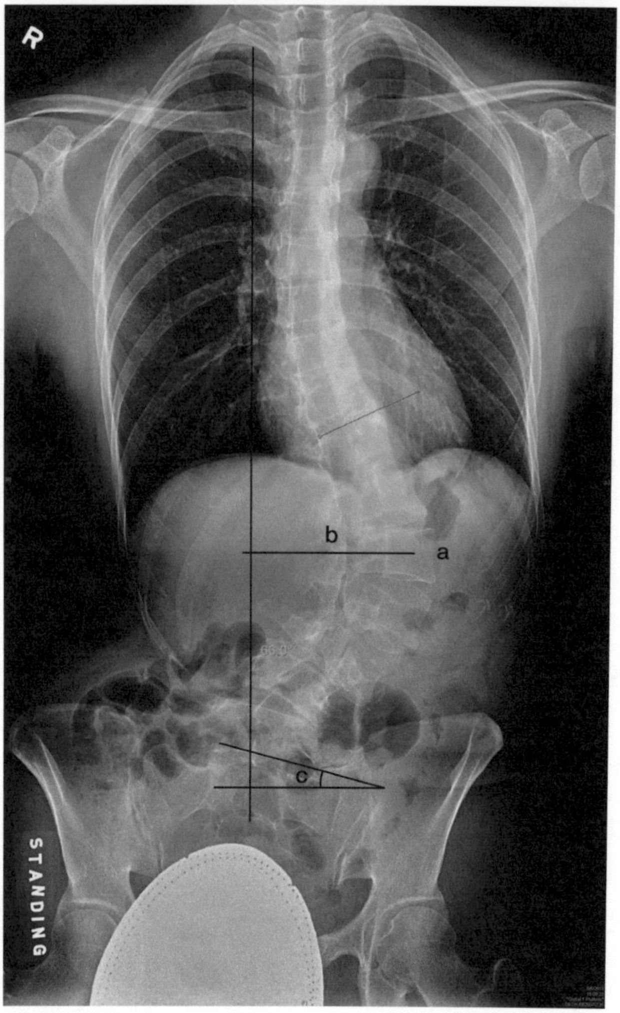

Figure 1.
The radiographic parameters that have been found to increase the risk of progression in adolescents with Lenke 5 and 6 scoliosis. It is likely that the parameters also increase the risk of curvature progression in adults. (a) Refers to the magnitude of apical vertebral rotation. (b) Refers to the distance between the central sacral line and the center of the apex of the lumbar curve. (c) Refers to the tilt angle of L5. When (a) is ≥III (based on the Nash-Moe method of measuring vertebral rotation), (b) is ≥4 cm, and (c) is ≥10°, the risk of progression of the curve increases.

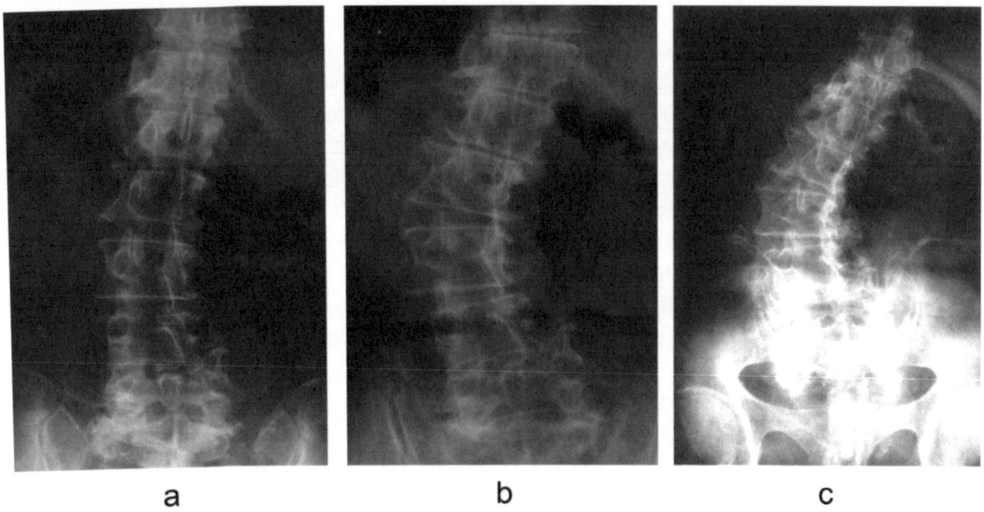

Figure 2.
The progression of degenerative lumbar scoliosis can be dramatic. The scoliosis in the frontal lumbar film of this woman 66 years of age was mild, with Cobb angle of 18° and the apex at L3 (a). The scoliosis progressed markedly 7 years later, with Cobb angle measuring 30°. Laterolisthesis of L1 to the right and L3 to the left could be seen (b). Arthrotic changes were apparent in the right in an attempt to stabilize the curvature, which, nevertheless, progressed to 44° 2 years later with marked rotation of L2–L4 vertebrae (c).

curves progressed 3° per year [13] and that apical vertebral rotation ≥ III (according to the Nash-Moe classification), a Cobb angle >30°, lateral vertebral translation >6 mm, and L5 above the intercristal line predict curve progression [13, 14]. Osteoporosis, a coronal Cobb angle <30°, lumbar lordosis, and degenerative spondylolisthesis are not risk factors for curve progression [14].

With increase in life expectancy of the population [2, 15], it follows that the prevalence of adult scoliosis increases [2, 15] and with it the morbidity.

2. Etiopathogenesis

There are many different causes of adult scoliosis. Majority of the adult scoliosis are adult idiopathic scoliosis (ADIS) and degenerative lumbar scoliosis (DLS). Other causes include neuromuscular conditions such as cerebral palsy, syringomyelia, and spinal dysraphism and congenital anomalies such as block vertebrae. Adult scoliosis may also arise from trauma, neoplastic disease, as well as iatrogenic causes such as simple decompression (laminectomy) or lumbar fusion procedures [16]. The following discussion will be limited to the commonly seen ADIS and DLS.

Idiopathic scoliosis, as its name implies, does not have any identifiable cause. When juveniles and adolescents who have idiopathic scoliosis reach adulthood or skeletal maturity, the scoliosis is then referred to as adult idiopathic scoliosis (ADIS).

The etiology of DLS is multifactorial and is related to progressive degeneration of the lumbar spine, compression fracture, and reduced bone density and quality [16]. The asymmetrical disc degeneration, facet degeneration, and ligamentous laxity all contribute to laxity in the spinal column [7, 17], with resultant asymmetrical deformities of the lumbar spine in the axial, coronal, and sagittal planes [18, 19]. The sagittal imbalance is accentuated in the presence of osteopenia or osteoporosis [16].

The mechanisms by which the scoliotic curves cause low back pain have not been clearly established. Pain can result from muscle overload, joint irritation, as well as nerve tension or compression. Initial complaints on the apex of the curvature are possibly a result of muscle overload, when the paravertebral muscles have to contract to maintain the spinal balance. With curve progression, joints become involved and the compressive, shear, and torsional forces concentrating in the concavity of the curve increase. Junctional segments are subjected to increased shear, favoring degenerative changes at these levels. When the shear force exerted on the junctional segments exceeds that of the restraining force, laterolisthesis may occur [20]. It is noteworthy that laterolisthesis is present even in mild lumbar scoliosis. In a study of 91 adults with lumbar idiopathic scoliosis, 9.75% of the patients were found to have laterolisthesis, despite the average lumbar Cobb angle being 16.5° [20]. The presence of lumbar laterolisthesis is associated with a higher frequency of back pain than do other curve patterns [10, 21]. When, however, osteophytes and traction spurs develop in those segments, the unstable segments may become stabilized with reduction in pain.

Depending on the level of involvement and anatomical configurations, nerve root entrapment may occur with radicular distress in the lower extremity. The nerve entrapment is usually present in the concavity of the curve, though it may also occur in the side of convexity. It is generally secondary to foraminal compression

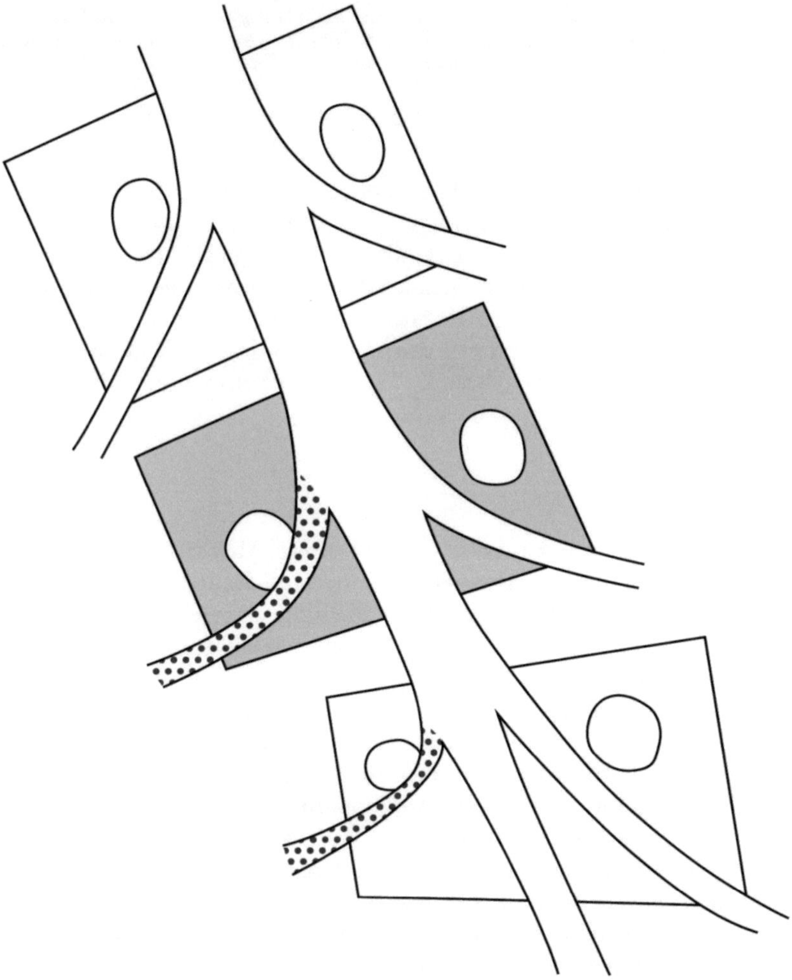

Figure 3.
The possible mechanism of nerve root entrapment in the concavity of the scoliotic curve. The laterolisthesis of the shaded vertebra to the left causes a downward migration of the left pedicle and exerts a pull on the nerve root. Owing to the lateral movement of the nerve root, the nerve root below is being stretched by the left pedicle. Thus a scoliosis can cause entrapment of nerve roots at two levels.

and pedicular kinking. With laterolisthesis, the pedicle migrates toward the side of concavity. The higher nerve root is thus stretched by the migrating pedicle (**Figure 3**); the lower nerve root similarly is stretched over the pedicle as it shifts laterally with the vertebral body above [22].

3. Clinical features

Many studies have shown that both ADIS and DLS may present with low back pain and radiculopathy. Yet, their characteristics differ [23]. ADIS patients usually have mechanical low back pain at an earlier age, at or around the age of 30. The pain is mechanical and seldom involves the leg [23].

In contrast, DLS patients have different pain patterns (**Table 1**). They are usually in the 50–60 years of age [24]. Those under 50 years of age with lumbar scoliosis are rarely subjected to significant pain and disability. Onset of the low back pain may be sudden but is usually progressive. Most commonly, the patient complains of low back pain at the end of a strenuous day or after some unusual activities. Rest reduces the pain. Pain is usually present at the apex of the curve, the lumbosacral junction, and the concavity of the scoliotic spine [25–27]. Very rarely is the pain brought about by impingement of the lower ribs upon the iliac crest [25].

	Degenerative lumbar scoliosis (DLS)	Adult idiopathic scoliosis (ADIS)
Age range at presentation (years)	55–57	25–56
Male/female incidence	41:59	4:96
Symptoms	Stenotic	Mechanical

Table 1.
The main difference in clinical presentation in patients with DLS and ADIS [24].

With progression of the condition, the patient may complain of radiating pain deep into the buttock and distally down the lower extremity, involving more than one dermatome with poorly defined boundaries [24]. Definite root entrapment is uncommon, and the incidence reported is 2.2% [26]. The severity of the complaint was found to be statistically significantly correlated with age. The older the patient, the more severe are the symptoms. A study of subjects over 50 years of age with DLS showed that 45 out of 200 patients (22.5%) had severe pain and neurological deficits [13].

3.1 Relationship between lumbar curve and low back pain

The relationship between the degree of lumbar curve and low back pain, however, has been controversial. Some authors [26, 27] reported that the greater the degree of scoliosis, the more is the pain. This is especially so for a curve that exceeds 45° [26]. In an analysis of pain pattern, Jackson and Simmons [27] found that the severity of low back pain varies with the level of scoliosis, the type of curve, and the degree of the curve. Lumbosacral, lumbar, and thoracolumbar curves were found to be more painful than thoracic curves. Comparing all curves, compensatory half curves are less painful, with one exception, viz., the left compensatory lumbosacral half curve. In the presence of a major and a compensatory curve, the pain usually localizes in the lower junctional segments and in the compensatory curve below the major deformity. In the presence of double major curves, however, the pain primarily affects the junctional areas below and between the major curves, with the lower one being more symptomatic [27].

Recent studies have shown that a coronal imbalance of more than 4–5 cm is associated with deterioration of pain and function scores in unoperated patients [28, 29]. Trunk shift is a predictor of surgery for patients with thoracolumbar and lumbar curvatures [29].

Yet, other authors did not concur with this view [9, 30]. They found no correlation between the degree of scoliosis and back symptoms. Lafage et al. reported no correlation between clinical outcomes and coronal global balance [30]; the magnitude of the coronal deformity did not impact pain and disability [30].

Recently, it has been shown that sagittal spinal balance is more important than coronal curves in relation to clinical outcomes [31–35]. The severity of the symptoms in adult scoliosis patients is linearly related to the magnitude of the sagittal spinal imbalance [36]. A spinal vertical axis (SVA) in excess of 70 mm is associated with an increase in clinical symptoms [30, 36].

4. Physical signs and physical examination

The patient usually walks with a typical antalgic list, with forward flexion of the spine and flexion of both knees. This is more evident as weakness with ambulation increases. Also, the patient is noted to sit obliquely, maintaining weight on one buttock and twisting away from the panful side [24]. Loss of height can occur. It was reported that a loss of height from 4 to 24 cm in 1–22 years may occur [37].

Examination in standing position permits assessment of the deformities as well as the sagittal and coronal imbalance. Adult scoliosis patients are often seen with trunk shift in the coronal plane together with positive sagittal imbalance. Reduction in lumbar lordosis is generally evident as the pelvis is retroverted to compensate for the positive sagittal malalignment. In severe deformity when the pelvic retroversion is insufficient to compensate for the sagittal imbalance, hip and knee flexion may be required to restore the sagittal balance. In the long term, contractures of hip flexors may result, when they can be assessed by Thomas leg raise test [38].

Inspection from the back may reveal the lumbar scoliosis. Generally, the pelvis shifts contralateral to the side of lumbar convexity. In the presence of left lumbar curvature, the pelvis shifts to the right and superiorly. The right pelvis is higher than the left. Conversely a right lumbar curvature is associated with shifting of the pelvis to the left [39]. This was confirmed by a study, which showed that 79% of patients with a single lumbar curve had the apex of the scoliosis opposite the side of high iliac crest [40]. The apparent leg length discrepancy that this created was reported in 87% of patients with degenerative lumbar scoliosis [40].

Assessment of the deformity may also be made in the sitting position to eliminate the confounding apparent leg length discrepancy or hip flexor contracture [38].

To determine the coronal balance, the distance from the gluteal cleft to a plumb line dropped from C7 is measured. When the head and trunk are not centered over the gluteal cleft and the measurement (coronal balance) is in excess of 4 cm, the scoliosis may be poorly compensated and more likely to progress [28].

Palpation may or may not elicit tenderness in the low back [9]. When tenderness is present, it is generally found in the concavity of the curve and at the junction between the two curves [27].

Neurological examination generally shows that there is reduced sensation in poorly defined areas. The reflexes of the lower extremities, however, are generally within normal limits. With increase in pain and disability, however, paresthesia over the posterolateral thigh and leg in areas of L5 and S1 dermatomal distribution becomes more evident, and reflexes in the lower extremities may reduce and become absent [41]. Straight leg raising is rarely restricted.

5. Clinical imaging

5.1 Radiography

Posteroanterior (PA) and lateral full spine radiographs are generally required. These enable assessment of global and regional spinopelvic alignment and assessment of the severity of the condition and the risk of curve progression.

To determine the coronal balance, a central sacral line (CSL) is drawn vertically from the center of the sacrum. The distance from C7 to the CSL is a measure of the coronal balance. From the PA film, the Cobb angle and the pelvic obliquity can also be determined. To measure the coronal Cobb angle, the upper and lower most tilted vertebrae (end vertebrae) are determined. Tangent lines are then drawn on the superior end plate of the upper end vertebra and the inferior end plate of the lower end vertebra, respectively. Perpendicular lines are then drawn to these two lines. The angle of intersection is the Cobb angle. The location of the curve is determined by the level of the apex, which is defined as the disc or vertebra maximally displaced from the midline and is minimally angulated. When the apex is located at T12 or L1, the curve is termed thoracolumbar curve; when the apex is inferior to L1, the curve is known as lumbar curve.

In DLS, the apex is generally located at the level of L2 and L3, with an associated distal fractional curve between L4 and S1. Compensatory curve when present is generally not structural and involves the thoracic and thoracolumbar areas [6]. Traction spurs and osteophytes are usually evident and are relatively large, situated on the concavity of the curve. Not uncommonly, laterolisthesis is present. In a long-term follow-up study, Weinstein and Ponseti [9] found that with time, marked translatory shift occurs between two vertebral segments in some lumbar and thoracolumbar curves. More severe structural deformities are characterized by laterolisthesis and rotatory subluxation, often at L3–L4 [20]. The shift took place at the lower end of the curve or at the transitional vertebra and is usually responsible for curve progression, which averages 3.3° in 10 years for both the thoracolumbar and lumbar curves [9, 20]. In mild curves with pelvic obliquity and more than 9 mm difference in hip levels, Giles and Taylor found an increased prevalence of L5 wedging in anteroposterior view, when compared with controls [42].

Vertebral rotation can be determined clinically using the Nash-Moe method or more accurately using the Raimondi or Perdriolle methods (**Figure 4**), both of which have low intra- and inter-observer errors [43–45]. The measurement is important as studies have shown that vertebral rotation >33% is associated with an increased incidence of back pain [9].

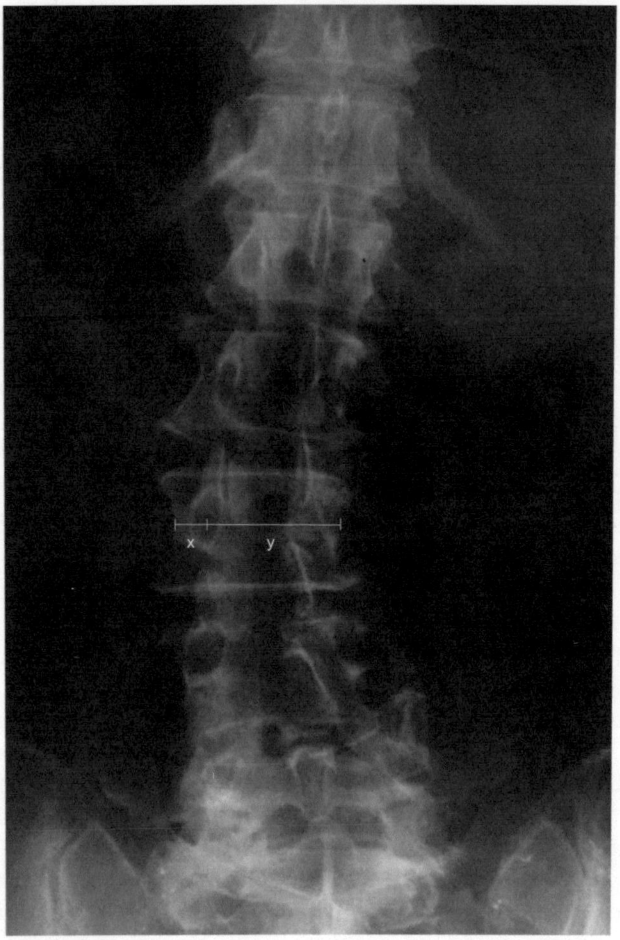

Figure 4.
Measurement of the apical vertebral rotation using the Raimondi method. The distance from the edge of the convex side of the apical vertebra to the center of the convex pedicle (x) is determined. The width of the vertebra (x + y) is then measured. From these two readings, the vertebral rotation can be determined using a Raimondi torsiometer.

Many recent studies have shown the importance of sagittal profile in relation to clinical outcome [30, 36, 46]. Many spinopelvic measurements have been found to correlate with the pain and disability. Schwab et al. showed that sagittal vertical axis (SVA), pelvic incidence minus lumbar lordosis, and pelvic tilt are related to disability and pain scores [46].

SVA is a measure of the sagittal imbalance. It is the horizontal distance between a vertical plumb line from the body of C7 to the posterosuperior corner of S1. The mean SVA of asymptomatic subjects was reported to be 0.5 ± 2.5 cm, whereas an ideal SVA was defined to be ±5 cm [47]. A SVA in excess of 7 cm was shown to be associated with an increase in clinical symptoms [36]. The findings were confirmed by other independent studies [30, 46]. Lafage et al. reported a correlation between the SVA and Scoliosis Research Society (SRS) total scores and Oswestry Disability Index (ODI) scores [30].

The SVA requires calibration of radiographs for measurement. To avoid the inherent error in measuring the offsets in non-calibrated radiographs, the T1 spinopelvic inclination (T1-SPI) angle may be used instead of SVA [30]. It is the angle subtended by a vertical plumb line from the center of T1 and a line drawn to bicoxofemoral axes (**Figure 5**). The angle has been shown to correlate with the health-related quality of life (HRQOL) scores [30]. Recently, Propopsalitis et al. (2014) proposed a novel radiographic measure of global spinal alignment, the T1 pelvic angle (TPA) [48]. It is the angle subtended by the lines connecting the bicoxofemoral axis to the center of T1 and the midpoint of the sacral end plate. Studies have shown that the measurement does not vary with pelvic retroversion or other postural compensatory mechanisms [48]. TPA was found to correlate with HRQOL scores. Treatment should attempt to reduce the TPA to <14°. Angle in excess of 20° corresponded to severe disability [48].

The pelvic incidence (PI) is also another important pelvic parameter that needs to be measured. It is a constant morphological parameter which has been shown to influence lumbar alignment. It is the angle subtended by the line connecting the midpoint of the bicoxofemoral axes and that of the sacral end plate and the perpendicular line to the latter. It should approximately match the lumbar lordosis (LL) (PI-LL = ±9°). A pelvic incidence-lumbar lordosis mismatch (PI-LL) in excess of 10° was reported to correlate with disability [46].

The PI is the sum of the pelvic tilt (PT) and sacral slope (SS) which are dynamic pelvic parameters that measure pelvic version, a compensatory mechanism to help maintain an upright posture in the setting of sagittal malalignment. The pelvic tilt is the angle subtended by the line connecting the midpoint of the bicoxofemoral

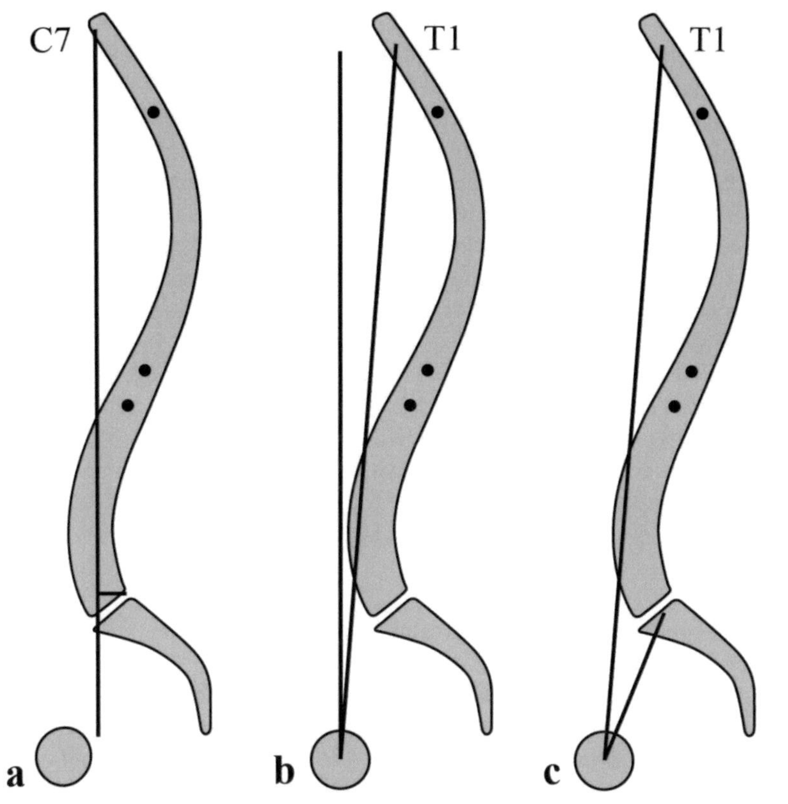

Figure 5.
The different methods of measuring global spinopelvic alignment. The sagittal vertical axis (a), the T1 spinopelvic inclination (T1-SPI) (b), and the T1 pelvic angle (TPA) (c).

axes and that of the sacral end plate and the vertical reference line extending upward from the femoral head axis. A positive sagittal imbalance as signified by an increased SVA is generally compensated by an increase in the pelvic tilt. A pelvic tilt of >22° is associated with disability [46].

5.2 Advanced imaging

In the presence of signs and findings of nerve root entrapment and intermittent claudication, referral for magnetic resonance imaging may be necessary to rule out the possibility of spinal cord impingement, spinal canal stenosis, lateral recess stenosis, or intraspinal lesions.

When osteoporosis is suspected, the patient should be referred for bone density assessment by dual-energy X-ray absorptiometry (DEXA) or the radiation-free echographic ultrasound [49], as reduction in bone density has been found to be lower in DLS patients when compared with normal controls with no scoliosis [5]. Also, bone mineral density (BMD) was found to correlate negatively with the scoliosis angle [50]. Furthermore, DLS patients with a lumbar curve in excess of 20° were found to have lower BMD than those with lumbar curves less than 20° [5].

6. Treatment

Treatment is generally conservative, particularly for patients who do not have rapidly progressive curves or significant neurological symptoms [6, 23, 51, 52]. Nonsteroidal anti-inflammatory drugs (NSAIDs), analgesics, manipulation, acupuncture, physiotherapy, and steroid injection were generally used to treat the low back pain and the accompanied radiculopathy [52, 53]. Outcome, however, was not satisfactory [52, 53]. A systematic review in 2007 showed that there was little evidence in support of these treatments in the management of adult scoliosis [52]. The studies identified level IV evidence for physical therapy, chiropractic care, and bracing and level III evidence for steroid injections [52]. Studies showed that the long-term successful rate of conservative treatment of symptomatic scoliosis was only 27% [33, 54].

The above treatments aim at pain reduction and stabilization of the curve, but not at the sagittal imbalance which is so often seen in patients with DLS. Recent studies have shown that physiotherapeutic scoliosis-specific exercises (PSSE), mirror image exercises, and chiropractic manipulation together with multimodal rehabilitation reduced pain and disability ratings in ADIS patients with thoracolumbar and lumbar curves [55–67]. Also, bracing is able to stabilize progressive curves in 80% of the adults with scoliosis [68].

6.1 Scoliosis-specific exercises and adult scoliosis

In the past 15 years, many different exercises and rehabilitation approaches to ADIS have been investigated. These include exercise, manipulation, and multimodal rehabilitation approaches [55–67, 69]. Exercises studied include yoga (side plank), Pilates, the side-shift and hitch exercise, the active self-correction, the Chiropractic BioPhysics® (CBP) mirror image, the FED, the Scientific Exercises Approach to Scoliosis (SEAS), and the Schroth Best Practice® (SBP®) program (**Table 2**). Other rehabilitation techniques investigated include the gravity traction, the weighting system, and manipulation [58, 62, 69]. These interventions have all been reported to reduce pain, disability, and the curves in ADIS.

Studies	Authors	No	Age	Types of scoliosis	Intervention	PI	Outcome
Case report/ series	Morningstar 2006 [26]	3	23–37	ADIS (TH)	Chiropractic and rehab	<12 weeks	Reduced curves (35 → 22°; 22 → 8°; 37 → 21°)
	Negrini 2008 [21]	1	25	ADIS (DM)	SEAS	1 year	Reduced curve (47 → 28.5°)
	Yang 2015 [22]	1	26	ADIS (TH)	Schroth + physio	8 weeks	Reduced curve (20.5 → 16.4°)
	Lebel 2016 [24]	1	23	ADIS (TH)	Schroth	More than 1 year	Reduced LBP and curve (70 → 58°; 48 → 43°)
	Harrison 2017 [18]	5	17–45	ADIS (TL or L)	CBP® + manipulation	18–84 visits	Reduced curves in 60%
	Haggard 2017 [25]	1	15	AIS (TL)	CBP® + manipulation	24 visits	Reduced LBP and curve after failure of chiropractic tx (27 → 8°)
Cohort	Barrios 2002 [15]	30	25–55	ADIS (MX)	FED device	20 = 60 sessions	Reduced back pain and curve (35 → 33°)
	Maruyama 2002 [17]	69	11–27	AIS and ADIS	Side shift and hitch	Mean 4.2 years	TL: (24.5 → 22.9°)
	Morningstar 2004 [20]	19	15–65	ADIS (MX)	Chiropractic and rehab	4–6 weeks	Reduced curve mean reduction 17°
	Morningstar 2011 [16]	28	18–54	ADIS (MX)	Chiropractic and rehab	6 months	Reduced curves and disability rating; TL (39.2 → 22°)
	Fishman 2014 [23]	25	14–85	ADIS; DLS (MX)	Side plank	3–22 months	Reduced 32% of the curve (37.2 → 25.3°)
	Negrini 2015 [13]	34	38 ± 11	ADIS (MX)	SEAS	2 years	Reduced curves in 69% TL (49 → 46°)
	Ng 2018 [19]	12	59 ± 15	ADIS and DLS	Schroth Best Practice	9 months	Reduced curves in 33%
RCT	Monticone 2016 [14]	130	51.6	ADIS (MX)	Self-correction and cognitive training	20 weeks	Reduced disability and curves

No, number of patients; PI, period of intervention; ADIS, adult patients with idiopathic scoliosis; DLS, degenerative lumbar scoliosis; MX, mixed curve types; TH, thoracic scoliosis; DM, double major curves; TL, thoracolumbar curve; L, lumbar curve; CBP®, chiropractic biophysics; SEAS, Scientific Exercises Approach to Scoliosis.

Table 2.
Studies on exercises and rehabilitation on the curves and pain in adult scoliosis patients.

6.1.1 Pain reduction

A number of studies have reported a reduction of pain after scoliosis-specific exercises intervention [60, 64]. Yang reported a reduction in pain in a young female with ADIS with a thoracic curvature using the SBP®, together with the standard physiotherapy care [64]; the pain scale (visual analogue scale, VAS) of the patient reduced from 5 to 1. Lebel and Lebel reported a severe case of thoracic scoliosis treated by Schroth exercises [66]. After 9 months of exercises, the thoracic curve of the 23-year-old female patient with adolescent idiopathic scoliosis reduced from 70 to 58° and the lumbar curve from 48 to 43° [66]. There was a significant reduction in low back pain after 1 month of exercise [66]. Harrison and Oakley reported similar findings in five ADIS with thoracolumbar or lumbar curves, using the CBP® mirror image method [60]. All the five cases reported a reduction of VAS, with the most significant one dropping from 6 to 0 [60]. The findings agreed with the results of a randomized controlled trial which showed that stabilization exercises which included active self-correction, task-oriented activities, and cognitive behavior therapy improved the Oswestry Disability Index (ODI) of ADIS when compared to standard physiotherapy treatment [56].

6.1.2 Cobb angle reduction

Many studies similarly showed that rehabilitation and specific exercises improve curves in ADIS and patients with DLS [58, 60, 61]. Some studies have shown that manipulation together with multimodal rehabilitation reduced scoliosis curves. In a retrospective review, Morningstar et al. showed that chiropractic treatment together with multimodal rehabilitation for 4–6 weeks reduced the curves in all of the 19 adult patients with idiopathic scoliosis [62]. This was confirmed by a subsequent study, which reported that 6 months of multimodal treatment together with manipulation reduced scoliosis curves and disability ratings in 28 ADIS aged 18–54 [58]. Non-specific exercises and physiotherapeutic scoliosis-specific exercises (PSSE) have also been found to improve curvatures in ADIS [55, 65, 66]. Fishman et al. reported that performance of side plank exercises daily for as long as tolerable (around 2 minutes) on the side of scoliosis convexity reduced the curves in ADIS and DLS patients [65]. Daily side plank exercises for 3–22 months reduced curves significantly in 30% of the adult scoliosis patients [65]. Yet, the study included adolescents aged 14 as well as patients with a Cobb angle less than 10°, which is strictly speaking not scoliosis [65]. Negrini et al. reported the outcome of SEAS intervention in a 25-year-old female adult with progressive double major curve, which progressed by 10° in 6 years [63]. In the follow-up 1 year later, the curvatures were found to reduce significantly from 47 to 28.5°. The authors attributed the positive change to an improvement in postural collapse [63]. The results were supported by a retrospective cohort study conducted by the same group [55]. SEAS intervention for 2 years resulted in an improvement of the Cobb angle in 68% of the 34 ADIS aged 38 ± 11 [55]. The mean reduction in the Cobb angle was 4.6 ± 5.0°, with no differences based on the location of the curve, gender, and length of treatment [55]. Monticone et al. compared the outcome of stabilization exercises using self-correction, task-oriented activities, and cognitive behavior therapy with standard physiotherapy care, which consisted of active and passive mobilizations, stretching, and strengthening exercises of the spinal muscles in the treatment of ADIS [56]. In the randomized controlled trial which involved 130 patients with a mean age of 51.6, they found that the experimental group had a reduced Cobb angle after 20 weeks of intervention as compared to the control group. Schroth exercises have also been found to reduce curves in adult scoliosis patients [64, 66]. Ng et al., in a prospective study, showed that home-based SBP® program for 9 months reduced the thoracolumbar or lumbar curvature in over 30% of the ADIS and DLS patients [61]. Harrison and Oakley reported the outcome of CBP® mirror image method in the treatment of thoracolumbar and lumbar curves in five patients with ADIS. In 18–84 visits, the treatment improved the curvatures in 60% of the patients, when a reduction of ≥6° is regarded as an improvement [60]. The CBP® mirror image method was regarded as similar to Schroth exercises [60].

6.1.3 Sagittal profile

While there were many studies addressing the coronal curves in ADIS and DLS patients, there were very few studies addressing the impact of PSSE on the sagittal profile of the patients [61]. The effects of PSSE on the sagittal profile of this group of patients are thus uncertain.

6.2 Other physical interventions

Hanging exercises should not be included as they have not been found useful [70]. Periodic axial spinal unloading using the LTX3000 lumbar rehabilitation system did not permanently affect the scoliosis; unloading of the spine temporarily reduced the scoliosis angle in adult scoliosis subjects, but with cessation of the intervention, the curves reverted back to the baseline level [70].

As thoracolumbar and lumbar curves are frequently associated with pelvic shift and obliquity, with secondary apparent leg length discrepancy, it is tempting to apply sole lift on the side of the low pelvis. Lehnert-Schroth advised against the use of sole lift. Addition of the sole lift on the side of the low pelvis would cause spinal imbalance, as evidenced by the tilted gluteal cleft [39]. Instead, patients should be advised to contract the hip abductor on the side of the higher pelvis to level the pelvis [39]. The patients can also flex the knee on the side of the high iliac crest [71] or raise the heel on the side of the low iliac crest when standing at ease [72]. This would reduce the lumbar curve and the associated stress on the facet joints and the adjoining soft tissue structures.

6.3 Spinal bracing

The effects of bracing in the treatment of adult scoliosis patients have been controversial [17, 68]. Some authors were of the opinion that brace does not halt curve progression and any pain relief provided is offset by associated deconditioning [7, 17]. Yet, recent studies have shown that spinal bracing stabilized the curves [68, 73, 74]. In a study which followed 158 adults with spinal deformities (ASD) treated by lordosing bivalve polyethylene overlapping brace for over 5 years showed that 24% of the curves reduced by more than 5°, 56% of the curves stabilized (±5°), and 20% worsened (>5°) [68]. Similarly, Palazzo et al. in a long-term follow-up study of 22 years showed that the progression of curves in ADIS and DLS patients reduced [74]. The yearly progression for curves in patients with DLS reduced from 1.47 to 0.24° per year and that for patients with ADIS from 0.7 to 0.24° per year [74]. de Mauroy suggested that the brace treatment is not only palliative; it treats lumbar instability by reducing the pressure in disc and stabilizing the lumbar area in lordosis [73].

7. Clinical management

Adult patients with low back pain and thoracolumbar and lumbar curves which have a high risk of progression or which are accompanied by sagittal imbalance are suggested to be treated by scoliosis-specific exercises, together with standard physiotherapy care. Exercises should target at improving the sagittal profile as well as the coronal curves. The exercises should preferably be supervised, as studies have shown that the physiotherapist-supervised Schroth Best Practice® (SBP®) exercises were associated with better outcome than home-based SBP® exercises [75]. In case of curve progression or pain, the patient should be prescribed a spinal brace. He or she should wear it 6–8 hours a day or as needed and perform the corrective scoliosis-specific exercises 3–4 times weekly to avoid deconditioning of the truncal muscles.

Recent studies showed that 46.6% of patients with DLS had sarcopenia involving the appendix and the trunk [76]. The trunk skeletal muscle mass index (SMI) was found to be significantly negatively correlated with SVA, PT, lumbar scoliosis, and apical vertebral rotation, suggesting that the reduction in trunk musculature was related to the stooped posture, pelvic retroversion, and lumbar scoliosis [76]. In view of the propensity of the DLS to progress, PSSE may also be taught to DLS patients who are asymptomatic as preventive measures.

If all these interventions fail and the patient has signs and symptoms suggestive of clinically significant spinal stenosis, he or she should be referred for surgical management [77].

Author details

Shu-Yan Ng[1], Tsz-Ki Ho[2]* and Yin-Ling Ng[2]

1 Wanchai Chiropractic Clinic, Wanchai, Hong Kong

2 Spine Technology Ltd, Wanchai, Hong Kong

*Address all correspondence to: angelh@ezped.com

References

[1] Kobayashi T, Atsuta Y, Takemitsu M, Matsuno T, Takeda N. A prospective study of de novo scoliosis in a community based cohort. Spine (Phila Pa 1976). 2006;**31**:178-182

[2] Urrutia J, Diaz-Ledezma C, Espinosa J, Berven SH. Lumbar scoliosis in postmenopausal women: Prevalence and relationship with bone density, age, and body mass index. Spine (Phila Pa 1976). 2011;**36**(9):737-740

[3] Kebaish KM, Neubauer PR, Voros GD, Khoshnevisan MA, Skolasky RL. Scoliosis in adults aged 40 years and older: Prevalence and relationship to age, race, and gender. Spine (Phila Pa 1976). 2011;**1976**:731-736

[4] Schwab F, Dubey A, Pagala M, Gamez L, Farcy JP. Adult scoliosis: A health assessment analysis by SF-36. Spine (Phila Pa 1976). 2003;**28**:602-606

[5] Xu L, Sun X, Huang S, Zhu Z, Qiao J, Zhu F, et al. Degenerative lumbar scoliosis in Chinese Han population: Prevalence and relationship to age, gender, bone mineral density, and body mass index. European Spine Journal. 2013;**22**(6):1326-1331

[6] Silva FE, Lenke LG. Adult degenerative scoliosis: Evaluation and management. Neurosurgical Focus. 2010;**28**(3):E1

[7] Pizones J, Martin-Buitrago MP, Perez-Grueso JS, et al. Function and clinical symptoms are main factors that motivate thoracolumbar adult scoliosis patients to pursue surgery. Spine (Phila Pa 1976). 1 Jan 2017;**42**(1):E31-E36

[8] Marty-Poumarat C, Scattin L, Marpeau M, Garreau de Loubresse C, Aegerter P. Natural history of progressive adult scoliosis. Spine. 2007;**32**(11):1227-1234

[9] Weinstein SL, Ponseti IV. Curve progression in idiopathic scoliosis. The Journal of Bone and Joint Surgery. American Volume. 1983;**65**(4):447-455

[10] Ascani E, Bartolozzi P, Logroscino CA, et al. Natural history of untreated idiopathic scoliosis after skeletal maturity. Spine (Phila Pa 1976). 1986;**11**(8):784-789

[11] Iida T, Ohyama Y, Katayanagi J, Ato A, Mine K, Matsumoto K, et al. Differences between pre-existing type and de novo type left convex thoracolumbar/lumbar scoliosis. Scoliosis. 2015;**10**(Suppl 2):S6

[12] Li Z, Li G, Chen C, Li Y, Yang C, Li M, et al. The radiographic parameter risk factors of rapid curve progression in Lenke 5 and 6 adolescent idiopathic scoliosis: A retrospective study. Medicine (Baltimore). 2017;**96**(52):e9425

[13] Pritchett JW, Bortel DT. Degenerative symptomatic lumbar scoliosis. Spine (Phila Pa 1976). 1993;**18**(6):700-703

[14] Faraj SS, Holewijn RM, van Hooff ML, de Kleuver M, Pellisé F, Haanstra TM. De novo degenerative lumbar scoliosis: A systematic review of prognostic factors for curve progression. European Spine Journal. 2016;**25**(8):2347-2358

[15] Jimbo S, Kobayashi T, Aono K, Atsuta Y, Matsuno T. Epidemiology of degenerative lumbar scoliosis: A community-based cohort study. Spine (Phila Pa 1976). 2012;**37**(20):1763-1770

[16] Yang C, Yang MY, Chen YY, Wei XZ, Ni HJ, Chen ZQ, et al. Radiographic parameters in adult degenerative scoliosis and different parameters between sagittal balanced and

imbalanced ads patients. Medicine (Baltimore). Jul 2015;**94**(29):e1198

[17] Youssef JA, Orndorff DO, Patty CA, et al. Current status of adult spinal deformity. Global Spine Journal. 2013;**3**(1):51-62

[18] Kotwal S, Pumberger M, Hughes A, et al. Degenerative scoliosis: A review. HSS Journal. 2011;7:257-264

[19] Tempel ZJ, Gandhoke GS, Bonfield CM, et al. Radiographic and clinical outcomes following combined lateral lumbar interbody fusion and posterior segmental stabilization in patients with adult degenerative scoliosis. Neurosurgical Focus. 2014;**36**:E11

[20] Korovessis P, Piperos G, Sidiropoulos P, Diures A. Adult idiopathic lumbar scoliosis. A formula for prediction of progression and review of the literature. Spine. 1994;**19**(17):1926-1932

[21] Weinstein SL, Dolan LA, Cheng JC, Danielsson A, Morcuende JA. Adolescent idiopathic scoliosis. Lancet. 2008;**371**(9623):1527-1537

[22] Simmons EH, Jackson RP. The management of nerve root entrapment syndromes associated with the collapsing scoliosis of idiopathic lumbar and thoracolumbar curves. Spine (Phila Pa 1976). 1979;**4**(6):533-541

[23] Grubb SA, Lipscomb HJ, Coonrad RW. Degenerative adult onset scoliosis. Spine (Phila Pa 1976). 1988;**13**(3):241-245

[24] San Martino A, D'Andria FM, San Martino C. The surgical treatment of nerve root compression caused by scoliosis of the lumbar spine. Spine (Phila Pa 1976). 1983;**8**(3):261-265

[25] Briard JL, Jegou D, Cauchoix J. Adult lumbar scoliosis. Spine (Phila Pa 1976). 1979;**4**(6):526-532

[26] Kostuik JP, Bentivoglio J. The incidence of low-back pain in adult scoliosis. Spine (Phila Pa 1976). 1981;**6**(3):268-273

[27] Jackson RP, Simmons EH, Stripinis D. Incidence and severity of back pain in adult idiopathic scoliosis. Spine (Phila Pa 1976). 1983;**8**(7):749-756

[28] Glassman SD, Berven S, Bridwell K, Horton W, Dimar JR. Correlation of radiographic parameters and clinical symptoms in adult scoliosis. Spine. 2005;**30**:682-688

[29] Ploumis A, Liu H, Mehbod AA, et al. A correlation of radiographic and functional measurements in adult degenerative scoliosis. Spine. 2009;**34**:1581-1584

[30] Lafage V, Schwab F, Patel A, Hawkinson N, Farcy JP. Pelvic tilt and truncal inclination: Two key radiographic parameters in the setting of adults with spinal deformity. Spine (Phila Pa 1976). 2009;**34**(17):E599-E606

[31] Mac-Thiong JM, Labelle H, Charlebois M, et al. Sagittal plane analysis of the spine and pelvis in adolescent idiopathic scoliosis according to the coronal curve type. Spine. 2003;**28**:1404-1409

[32] Li WS, Li G, Chen ZQ, et al. Sagittal plane analysis of the spine and pelvis in adult idiopathic scoliosis. Chinese Medical Journal. 2010;**123**:2978-2982

[33] Savage JW, Patel AA. Fixed sagittal plane imbalance. Global Spine Journal. 2014;**4**:287-296

[34] Lazennec JY, Ramare S, Arafati N, et al. Sagittal alignment in lumbosacral fusion: Relations between radiological parameters and pain. European Spine Journal. 2000;**9**:47-55

[35] Schwab F, Ungar B, Blondel B, et al. Scoliosis Research Society-Schwab adult spinal deformity

classification: A validation study. Spine. 2012;**37**:1077-1082

[36] Glassman SD, Bridwell K, Dimar JR, Horton W, Berven S, Schwab F. The impact of positive sagittal balance in adult spinal deformity. Spine. 2005;**30**(18):2024-2029

[37] Stagnara P. Scoliosis in adults. Consequences of idiopathic scoliosis in adulthood. Chirurgie. 1982;**108**(4):356-363

[38] Ames CP, Smith JS, Scheer JK, et al. Impact of spinopelvic alignment on decision making in deformity surgery in adults: A review. Journal of Neurosurgery: Spine. 2012;**16**(6):547-564

[39] Lehnert Schroth C. Three-dimensional treatment for scoliosis. A physiotherapeutic method for deformities of the spine. Calif: Martindale Press; 2007

[40] Radcliff KE, Orozco F, Molby N, Chen E, Sidhu GS, Vaccaro AR, et al. Is pelvic obliquity related to degenerative scoliosis? Orthopaedic Surgery. 2013;**5**(3):171-176

[41] Smith JS, Shaffrey CI, Fu KM, et al. Clinical and radiographic evaluation of the adult spinal deformity patient. Neurosurgery Clinics of North America. 2013;**24**(2):143-156

[42] Giles LG, Taylor JR. Low-back pain associated with leg length inequality. Spine (Phila Pa 1976). 1981;**6**(5):510-521

[43] Weiss HR. Measurement of vertebral rotation: Perdriolle versus Raimondi. European Spine Journal. 1995;**4**(1):34-38

[44] Barsanti CM, DeBari A, Covino BM. The torsion meter: A critical review. Journal of Pediatric Orthopaedics. 1990;**10**:527-531

[45] Omeroglu H, Ozekin O, Bicimoglu A. Measurement of vertebral rotation in idiopathic scoliosis using the Perdriolle torsionmeter: A clinical study on intraobserver and interobserver error. European Spine Journal. 1996;**5**:167-171

[46] Schwab FJ, Blondel B, Bess S, Hostin R, Shaffrey CI, et al. Radiographical spinopelvic parameters and disability in the setting of adult spinal deformity: A prospective multicenter analysis. Spine (Phila Pa 1976). 2013;**38**(13):E803-E812

[47] Jackson RP, McManus AC. Radiographic analysis of sagittal plane alignment and balance in standing volunteers and patients with low back pain matched for age, sex, and size. A prospective controlled clinical study. Spine (Phila Pa 1976). 1994;**19**(14):1611-1618

[48] Protopsaltis TS, Lafage R, Smith JS, Passias PG, Shaffrey CI, Kim HJ, et al. International spine study group. The lumbar pelvic angle, the lumbar component of the T1 pelvic angle, correlates with HRQOL, PI-LL mismatch, and it predicts global alignment. Spine (Phila Pa 1976). 2018;**43**(10):681-687

[49] Casciaro S, Conversano F, Pisani F, Muratore M. New perspectives in echographic diagnosis of osteoporosis on hip and spine. Clinical Cases in Mineral and Bone Metabolism. 2015;**12**(2):142-150

[50] Ding WY, Yang DL, Cao LZ, Sun YP, Zhang W, Xu JX, et al. Intervertebral disc degeneration and bone density in degenerative lumbar scoliosis: A comparative study between patients with degenerative lumbar scoliosis and patients with lumbar stenosis. Chinese Medical Journal. 2011;**124**(23):3875-3878

[51] Birknes JK, Harrop JS, White AP, Albert TJ. Adult degenerative scoliosis: A review. Neurosurgery. 2008;**63**(3 suppl):94-103

[52] Everett CR, Patel RK. A systematic literature review of nonsurgical treatment in adult scoliosis. Spine (Phila Pa 1976). 2007;**32**(19 suppl):S130-S134

[53] Kluba T, Dikmenli G, Dietz K, Giehl JP, Niemeyer T. Comparison of surgical and conservative treatment for degenerative lumbar scoliosis. Archives of Orthopaedic and Traumatic Surgery. 2009;**129**:1-5

[54] Ryan DJ, Protopsaltis TS, Ames CP, Hostin R, Klineberg E, Mundis GM, et al. International spine study group. T1 pelvic angle (TPA) effectively evaluates sagittal deformity and assesses radiographical surgical outcomes longitudinally. Spine (Phila Pa 1976). 2014;**39**(15):1203-1210

[55] Negrini A, Negrini MG, Donzelli S, Romano M, Zaina F, Negrini S. Scoliosis-Specific exercises can reduce the progression of severe curves in adult idiopathic scoliosis: A long-term cohort study. Scoliosis. 2015;**10**:20

[56] Monticone M, Ambrosini E, Cazzaniga D, Rocca B, Motta L, Cerri C, et al. Adults with idiopathic scoliosis improve disability after motor and cognitive rehabilitation: Results of a randomised controlled trial. European Spine Journal. 2016;**25**(10):3120-3129

[57] Barrios C, Lapuente JP, Sastre S. Treatment of chronic pain in adult scoliosis. Studies in Health Technology and Informatics. 2002;**88**:290-303

[58] Morningstar MW. Outcomes for adult scoliosis patients receiving chiropractic rehabilitation: A 24-month retrospective analysis. Journal of Chiropractic Medicine. 2011;**10**:179-178

[59] Maruyama T, Kitagawal T, Takeshita K, Nakainura K. Side shift exercise for idiopathic scoliosis after skeletal maturity. Studies in Health Technology and Informatics. 2002;**91**:361-364

[60] Harrison DE, Oakley PA. Scoliosis deformity reduction in adults: A CBP® Mirror Image case series incorporating the 'non-commutative property of finite rotation angles under addition' in five patients with lumbar and thoraco-lumbar scoliosis. Journal of Physical Therapy Science. 2017;**29**(11):2044-2050

[61] Ng SY, Chan WY, Ho TK, Ng YL. A pilot study on the effect of outpatient Schroth exercises on thoracolumbar and lumbar curves in adult scoliosis patients. In: Bettany-Saltikov J, Schreiber S, editors. Innovations in Spinal Deformities and Postural Disorders. Rijeka: Intech; 2017. pp. 93-112

[62] Morningstar MW, Woggon D, Lawrence G. Scoliosis treatment using a combination of manipulative and rehabilitative therapy: A retrospective case series. BMC Musculoskeletal Disorders. 2004;**5**:32

[63] Negrini A, Parzini S, Negrini MG, Romano M, Atanasio S, Zaina F, et al. Adult scoliosis can be reduced through specific SEAS exercises: A case report. Scoliosis. 2008;**3**:20

[64] Yang JM, Lee JH, Lee DH. Effects of consecutive application of stretching, Schroth, and strengthening exercises on Cobb's angle and the rib hump in an adult with idiopathic scoliosis. Journal of Physical Therapy Science. 2015;**27**(8):2667-2669

[65] Fishman LM, Groessl EJ, Sherman KJ. Serial case reporting yoga for idiopathic and degenerative scoliosis. Global Advances in Health and Medicine. 2014;**3**(5):16-21

[66] Lebel A, Lebel VA. Severe progressive scoliosis in an adult female possibly secondary thoracic surgery in childhood treated with scoliosis specific Schroth physiotherapy: Case presentation. Scoliosis and Spinal Disorders. 2016;**11**(Suppl 2):41

[67] Haggard JS, Haggard JB, Oakley PA, Harrison DE. Reduction of progressive thoracolumbar adolescent idiopathic scoliosis by chiropractic biophysics® (CBP®) mirror image® methods following failed traditional chiropractic treatment: A case report. Journal of Physical Therapy Science. 2017;**29**(11):2062-2067

[68] de Mauroy JC, Lecante C, Barral F, Pourret S. Prospective study of 158 adult scoliosis treated by a bivalve polyethylene overlapping brace and reviewed at least 5 years after brace fitting. Scoliosis and Spinal Disorders. 2016;**11**(Suppl 2):28

[69] Morningstar MW, Joy T. Scoliosis treatment using spinal manipulation and the Pettibon Weighting System TM: A summary of 3 typical presentations. Chiropractic and Osteopathy. 2006;**14**:1

[70] Hales J, Larson P, Iaizzo PA. Treatment of adult lumbar scoliosis with axial spinal unloading using the LTX3000 lumbar rehabilitation system. Spine. 2002;**27**(3):E71-E79

[71] Weiss HR, Lehnert-Schroth C, Moramarco M. Schroth Therapy: Advances in Conservative Scoliosis Treatment. Germany: Lap Lambert Acad Pub; 2015

[72] Maruyama T, Takeshita K, Kitagawa T. Side-shift exercise and hitch exercise. Studies in Health Technology and Informatics. 2008;**135**:246-249

[73] de Mauroy JC, Lecante C, Barral F, Pourret S. Bracing in adult with scoliosis: Experience in diagnosis and classification from a 15 year prospective study of 739 patients. Scoliosis and Spinal Disorders. 2016;**11**(Suppl 2):29

[74] Palazzo C, Montigny JP, Barbot F, Bussel B, Vaugier I, Fort D, et al. Effects of bracing in adult with Scoliosis: A retrospective study. Archives of Physical Medicine and Rehabilitation. 2017;**98**:187-190

[75] Kuru T, Yeldan İ, Dereli EE, Özdinçler AR, Dikici F, Çolak İ. The efficacy of three-dimensional Schroth exercises in adolescent idiopathic scoliosis: A randomised controlled clinical trial. Clinical Rehabilitation. 2016;**30**(2):181-190

[76] Eguchi Y, Suzuki M, Yamanaka H, Tamai H, Kobayashi T, Orita S, et al. Associations between sarcopenia and degenerative lumbar scoliosis in older women. Scoliosis and Spinal Disorders. 2017;**12**:9

[77] Neuman BJ, Baldus C, Zebala LP, Kelly MP, Shaffrey C, et al. Patient factors that influence decision making: Randomization versus observational nonoperative versus observational operative treatment for adult symptomatic lumbar scoliosis (ASLS). Spine (Phila Pa 1976). 2016;**41**(6):E349-E358